Handbook for True Democracy

*How the Grassroots Can Create a Nation
Of, By and For All the People Through the Evolution
of Individual and Organizational Behavior*

John G. Mentzos, PhD
Illustration by Victor Guiza

U.R.R. Publishing

Handbook for True Democracy
How the Grassroots Can Create a Nation Of, By and For All the People
Through the Evolution of Individual and Organizational Behavior
All Rights Reserved.
Copyright © 2020 John G. Mentzos, PhD
v6.0

The opinions expressed in this manuscript are solely the opinions of the author and do not represent the opinions or thoughts of the publisher. The author has represented and warranted full ownership and/or legal right to publish all the materials in this book.

This book may not be reproduced, transmitted, or stored in whole or in part by any means, including graphic, electronic, or mechanical without the express written consent of the publisher except in the case of brief quotations embodied in critical articles and reviews.

U.R.R. Publishing

ISBN: 978-0-578-22786-3

Cover Illustration by Victor Guiza © 2020 Outskirts Press, Inc. All rights reserved - used with permission.

PRINTED IN THE UNITED STATES OF AMERICA

Nothing under heaven is more yielding than water;
But when it attacks things hard and resistant,
There is not one of them that can prevail.
That the yielding conquers the resistant
And the soft conquers the hard
Is a fact known by all men,
But utilized by none.

—*Tao Te Ching*

Table of Contents

Foreword i
Introduction iii
1. The Evolution in Our Political Revolution 1
2. Genocide and the Corporate Colonization of America 19
3. The Robber Barons 2.0 40
4. The Myth of the All-Powerful Corporate Oligarchy 48
5. Out of Darkness Comes Light 54
6. Centering the Conscious Mind 61
7. Centering the Heart 78
8. Balancing the Heart with the Mind 91
9. Centering the Systems of the Body 104
10. Eating to Center the Systems of the Self 116
11. You Are the DNA of Democracy 131
12. Formally Organizing Humanity for Healthy Democracy 146
13. The Reciprocal–Altruistic Sector of Society: Fertile Soil
    for Healthy Democracy? 157
14. Healthy Democracy as Organizational Culture 172
15. Theory of Healthy Democracy in Not-for-Profit Organization ... 192
16. Spreading the Healthy Democracy Meme throughout
    the Systems of Society 198
17. Tomorrow Morning 211
References 217
Bibliography 224

Foreword

DEMOCRACY IS NOT just a set of laws and a government structure it's a collective consciousness. The collective consciousness of democracy arises out of human nature when called forth by group psychology and the social constructs and cultural artifacts of a nation. The appropriate collective consciousness for an effective democracy is one that yields culture and process that manages human diversity in equitable ways. But group psychology and the social constructs of a nation can serve as a countervailing force to effective democracy as well. To the extent that such elements create consciousness focused on producing inequity and perpetuating the conflicts that arise out of human diversity, the public consciousness needed for true democracy is lost.

Handbook For True Democracy: How the Grassroots Can Create a Nation Of, By and For All the People Through the Evolution of Individual and Organizational Behavior is the culmination of the author's life's work on issues posed by human diversity, organizational culture and democratic process. It brings together new writings and updated theoretical foundations from previous articles and books by the author in a comprehensive view of the world pertinent to today's struggle to achieve authentic democracy. *Handbook For True Democracy* demonstrates how the evolution of culture can take place and how culture can create an environment that encourages grassroots participation in shaping the institutions of society. It is a guide for both individual and collective action that directly and indirectly challenges corporate oligarchy at the roots of its power, and a reference for developing a new consciousness in our nation that supports democracy for all.

on how to respond. But there is also uneasiness and division among traditional conservatives.

We have our everyday lives to live. But many feel that life as usual just doesn't apply as it once did. There is a vacuum. In part, this book addresses that vacuum by encouraging a deep breath of wellness to clear our collective consciousness and help us gain footing to move forward. It will take a thoughtful look at healthy grassroots democracy—how grassroots democracy offers hope and how healthy democracy can be cultivated throughout society despite these new developments.

In this book, wellness is approached, in part, through the lens of healthy democracy, and the subject of democracy is approached from the individual behavior and organizational behavior perspectives. *Handbook For True Democracy* is not about the Democrats vs. Republicans, whites vs. people of color, women vs. men, or Christians vs. Muslims, and at its core it's not even about the rich vs. the poor, although all those seemingly countervailing forces are implicated. First and foremost, this book is a work in support of healthy democracy—the democracy within our hearts, hands, and minds—waiting to be born in our lives, organizations, communities, and nation.

This country was founded on the ideals of democracy, but the benefits of those ideals were extended to only a selected few, a privileged class. The current administration appears to support a return to that original version. The Trump–Pence era is about continuing what both political parties are guilty of—the dismantling of the structures that encourage authentic democratic opportunities for all. So by my voicing the need for a healthy democracy, I am not advocating for what we had in the past or propping up either of our political parties. Instead, what I explore is a strategy for achieving what we the people could have if we *will* it to be: a remarkably healthy population, living in a profoundly democratic nation—an America greater than ever.

CHAPTER 1

The Evolution in Our Political Revolution

HUMANITY HAS BEEN engaged in a battle ever since the earliest of societies. It is political and psychological and even biological. It is also spiritual. We see it described in ancient lore and religious texts the world over, and now the battle appears to be reaching a critical point. Humanity is at an evolutionary crossroads. Our entire civilization and all higher life on Earth are at stake. It has been thousands of years in the making, but now we must choose between two radically different futures.

All life has organized itself through biological evolution, humanity included. But there is nothing more central to the survival of human civilization than our *psychological* evolution. The battle is between two radically different views of how humanity should be organized psychologically—and therefore culturally, politically, and spiritually. Evolutionary psychology frames this dilemma. Evolutionary psychology relies heavily on the theory of natural selection to explain the origins of human behavior. It is founded on the belief that biological adaptation and psychological adaptation are not qualitatively different from one another.

One of the leading proponents of evolutionary psychology is Richard Dawkins, the author of *The Selfish Gene* (1989). In this groundbreaking book, he explained that evolution began with what he calls a replicator. Replicators, according to Dawkins, came into existence while life existed in the "primordial soup." He said, "The replicator was the first set of molecules that could create copies of itself, thus launching the process of natural selection" (15).

The next evolutionary leap was the emergence of the gene. Dawkins asserted that while there is no universally agreed definition of a gene, his own working definition came from G. C. Williams, who called it "any portion of chromosomal material that potentially lasts for enough generations to serve as a unit of natural selection." Dawkins went on to associate genes with his idea of replicators that "a gene is a replicator with high copying-fidelity" (Dawkins 1989, 28).

Dawkins said that genes are the basic propagators of procreation—specifically, their own. Genes in the gene pool associate to create what Dawkins called "survival machines." Survival machines are any life form comprised of genes. The purpose of survival machines is to assist in the passing on of the genes to future generations through survival and procreation. Biological organisms from amoebas to human beings could be said to be programmed by genes "to survive and to reproduce" (Dawkins 1989, 88) for the sake of the genes. This includes, to some significant degree, other survival machines with the same genes, such as offspring or siblings.

Dawkins described features created genetically to deal with an unpredictable environment, such as controlling protein synthesis and building a capacity for learning and imagination, including the ability to simulate the future and consequently prepare for it. Another critical feature is the ability to mimic. He used the example of edible bugs developing, through evolution, the appearance of other bugs that taste bad to predators (Dawkins 1989, 64). He described behaviors among birds and other animals that misrepresent the facts of their situations (i.e., lie) to both predators and parents (65). These features have evolved to respond effectively to a hostile environment.

Dawkins asserted that survival machines view other survival machines not closely related to them genetically as merely a part of the environment, "something that gets in the way or to be exploited"

(Dawkins 1989, 66). Genes that use their environment most effectively win at the game of natural selection. The success of a gene is evident not only in its ability to procreate, but more importantly, in its ability to develop an *evolutionarily stable strategy*. According to Dawkins,

> A "strategy" is a preprogrammed behavioral policy. An example of a strategy is: "Attack opponent; if he flees pursue him; if he retaliates run away." ... ESS is defined as a strategy which, if most members of a population adopt it, cannot be bettered by an alternative strategy. (69)

Interestingly enough, after spending the lion's share of *The Selfish Gene* describing the selfishness of evolution, Dawkins suggested that measured altruism might sometimes be the best survival strategy. ESS strategies include cooperation not only among genes and relatives, but also among nonrelatives and between different species. Dawkins concluded that these incidents of cooperation, too, are due to the selfish gene. He asserted that most, if not all, seemingly altruistic behaviors have selfish genetic motives behind them. As for those that do not, most are likely due to what he called "misfires" (Dawkins 1989, 73).

According to Dawkins, another apparent expression of altruism occurs among animals that resemble each other. That is, animals that look like each other are more apt to behave in ways that appeared altruistic, e.g., more likely to protect the offspring of a look-alike animal. In a roundabout way, this might help to extend common genes into future generations. Dawkins suggested that this phenomenon might, in part, inspire racism (Dawkins 1989, 100).

Also described in *The Selfish Gene* was reciprocal altruism, which Dawkins defined by describing the relationship between the cleaner fish and larger fish. The smaller cleaner fish feeds on the parasites of the larger fish. The larger fish, which would normally eat the fish the size of a cleaner fish, refrains from eating fish with the cleaner fish markings (Dawkins 1989, 187). The relationship is a win-win called Tit-for-Tat. Dawkins said, "Tit-for-Tat begins by cooperating on the first move and thereafter simply copies the previous move of the other player" (Dawkins 1989, 210). He noted that Axelrod identified some key characteristics of winning strategies in the game. The first two were described as *nice* and *forgiving*.

> A nice strategy is defined as one that is never the first to defect. Tit-for-Tat is an example . . . A forgiving strategy is one that, although it may retaliate, has a short memory. It is swift to overlook old misdeeds. (Dawkins 1989, 212)

A third characteristic was *non-envious*:

> Tit-for-Tat is also non-envious. To be non-envious, in Axelrod's terminology, means not to strive for more money than the other player, rather for an absolutely large quantity of the banker's money. (Dawkins 1989, 220)

Dawkins said that the obvious insight provided by Tit-for-Tat-like strategy was that in the Prisoner's Dilemma involving multiple strategies, non-zero-sum games prevailed. The optimum result for both players was a win-win outcome. Dawkins described how Axelrod ran the experiment again using sixty-three strategies. Initially, strategies battled back and forth with fortunes rising and falling. It took about 1,000 generations to reach stability. That is, no further changes in the climate were found. Dawkins concluded that the " . . . tit-for-tat-like strategies were roughly equivalent to ESS in practice" (Dawkins 1989, 217). He seemed to suggest that Axelrod's computer experiments offered promise for win-win strategies in terms of evolution, not only in general, but particularly for humankind.

Tit-for-Tat experiments continued, eventually leading to Tit-for-Tat with forgiveness[1] prevailing as long as there are other Tit-for-Tat with

---

1   See Worthington 2004 on effect of forgiveness in society.

forgiveness players (Sapolsky 2005). For Dawkins, there was first the primordial soup with replicators (Dawkins 1989, 47–48); the gene pool (26); and most recently, the soup of human culture (192), containing the equivalent to the gene/replicator that Dawkins called the meme. Examples of meme offered by Dawkins (1989, 192) include:

> ...Tunes, ideas, catch phrases, clothing, fashions, ways of making pots or building arches. Just as genes propagate themselves in the gene pool by leaping from body to body via sperm or eggs, so memes propagate themselves in the meme pool by leaping from brain to brain via a process that, in the broad sense, can be called imitation.

Dawkins also suggested that memes, like genes, might compete with each other for dominance. According to his thesis, genes and memes are responsible for what many call sin, redemption, and virtue in humankind. Through biology and culture, humankind evolved for the sake of successfully passing on the genes and memes of which humans are comprised. So long as it pays to lie, be envious, murder, humanity is compelled to pursue just that. But when forgiveness, non-enviousness, and cooperation are more successful behaviors for pursuing those ends, virtue becomes the methodology in pursuit of the goal of humankind.

He noted that memes evolve at a much faster rate than genes do. They have the potential to quickly transform human behavior. As we have seen in the Prisoner's Dilemma experiment, altruism in measured amounts could be a successful strategy for evolution; the potential to evolve more altruistically exists. Thus, Dawkins implied, through culture humanity could, comparatively speaking, rapidly evolve toward a more altruistic world.

In his book *Evolution of the Mind* (2003), Richard Townsend conjectured about the biological origins of sin, redemption, and virtue, just as Dawkins did. Townsend framed evolution of the mind as the development of the human nervous system and brain through natural selection. The earliest phase of this development is the part of the nervous system that focuses on hunger (the impulse to feed) and procreation (15-17). Townsend called this mind the *primordial mind* (24). This portion of the mind also controls automatic body functions, e.g., the beating of the heart.

As the species developed, according to Townsend, the environment required the human mind to adapt to eat or be eaten. In this second phase of the evolution of the human mind, fear, deception, aggression (killing instinct), cunning, greed, hatred, and viciousness developed. Townsend called this addition to the mind the *animal mind* (Townsend 2003, 24). These attributes helped humanity to solve problems specific to survival and procreation in a hostile environment.

The final step, according to Townsend, was the emergence of the *social mind*. The social mind evolved to express love, compassion, cooperation, and respect, among other attributes. This portion of the mind evolved to succeed in environments that require groups of humans to work together in order to survive (Townsend 2003, 25). The act of conforming to the norms of the group is governed by the social mind, as is the desire to change others or banish them from the group (57).

Townsend discussed the aspects of the mind as if they are separate and often in conflict. Although this works well as a metaphor, in actuality the brain is a more integrated organ than the metaphor suggests. Nonetheless, according to Townsend, the impulse of the primordial and animal minds (presocial minds) has a tendency to conflict with the requirements of the social mind. "The conflicts between the presocial and social minds and their resolution," Townsend stated, "are the basis of ethics and morality. They are also basics of religion, psychology, and the law" (Townsend 2003, 62). Townsend expounded on the process as he saw it:

> The social mind uses two preprogrammed methods to control the presocial mind's action and the deportment of members of

> the social unit. On the one hand, the social mind uses shame, guilt, and disapproval as a control mechanism. The traits of shame, guilt, and the fear of disapproval are preprogrammed into the mind. They are very strong traits. Individual members attempt to conform to escape the pain and discomfort these traits impose. The other preprogrammed control mechanism is approval. Individuals function to gain the approval that comes from acting in a socially acceptable manner. . . . The rules of a society are passed down from generation to generation through individual contact. They are passed through education, the law, and religion. They are passed through psychology. They are passed through the written and spoken word, and through music and art. The attempt to escape shame, guilt, and disapproval, along with the attempt to gain approval, drives individual members of the social unit to adhere to these social guidelines. (67-68)

Townsend equated the attributes of the presocial minds with sin and the attributes of the social mind with redemption and virtue. The struggle between sin and virtue, according to Townsend, is the conflict between the presocial and social minds. Ultimately he equated the attributes of the presocial and social minds to the Devil and God, respectively.

> If we look at the attributes of the primordial and animal minds, we find, with the possible exception of hunger, that they are also the attributes ascribed to the Devil of religious lore. If we examine that concept of the Devil, we find the following attributes: He is deceptive. He is murderous. He is treacherous. He offers humankind emotional and sexual temptation as an inducement to fulfill his treacherous greed . . . If we examine the concept of God as defined by religious lore, we find that God has the following attributes: God is good. God is kind. God is loving. God is considerate. God is compassionate.

argued that what seem to be altruistic acts in nature are usually misfires—that is, they are accidents or at best temporary cooperation that he called "pacts and conspiracies to further selfish aspirations." Dawkins has essentially argued against the idea that evolution is motivated by altruism. Nonetheless, evolutionary impulses could pursue reciprocal-altruistic arrangements if a more successful dissemination of genes or memes resulted. Reciprocal altruism could potentially lead to the common good between individuals who otherwise would be competitive. Assuming Townsend is correct about a drive among the population toward social colonization and Dawkins is correct about the selfishness of evolution, then the social colonizers are more likely pursuing a reciprocal altruistic survival strategy rather than outright altruism.

Townsend argument that there is a struggle between divergent evolutionary strategies to shape future society, in essence, frames the underlying culture war in America. The winner of this struggle will determine the evolution of human psychology and consequently the future of human culture, politics, and spirituality. In Townsend's view, this is a struggle between colonizers and individualists opposed to colonization. But this can't be a truly contested struggle comprising unaffiliated individuals versus a society of colonizers of course. Without counter organization, the individualist or many unconnected and independent individualists are no contest against an entire committed society. The resources and numbers of people in society would always overcome the lone wolf, even if the lone wolf, pound for pound, were stronger and more cunning than the average member of the pack or colony.

In order for the lone individualist to successfully challenge a society moving toward colonization, that person would have to use their superior cunning and deceit to manipulate the environment on a scale large enough to serve his or her countervailing agenda. The individualists at some point must connect to a unifying organizing principle in order to compete with a society evolving toward social mind colonization. Organizing principles such as capitalism and imperialism could help achieve this because both allow the most successful among individualists to accumulate enough resources to affect the environment of society. For example, individuals who can establish militaries can pursue imperialism. Imperialism exists to control societies through force and guile in order to usurp resources for the benefit of highly successful individualists, even at the expense of millions of people. If the resources achieved through capitalism were immense enough, these profits could in turn be used to co-opt leadership and the institutions that they control, and this process could be used to influence the society of colonizers to create structures that benefit highly successful individualists. What I am suggesting is that it is more likely that a class of highly successful individualists in cooperation has and continues to emerge throughout history. These super successful individualists are (in affect) *super successful* Cheats (to build on the Dawkins analogy of evolutionary strategies). This class of individualists, in cooperation with each other, is more likely to be the primary countervailing force to social mind colonization because of their motives, cultural orientation and organizational capacity.

This struggle between evolutionary strategies is a battle between which form of colonization will prevail. On one side of this battle there is the colonization driven by highly dominant individualists (Super Cheats) in cooperation: the *Few* (i.e., oligarchy of economic elite primarily oriented by the presocial minds and the culture that's supportive of them). On the other side of this struggle is the colonization that arises out of *the many:* less-dominant *mutualists* (reciprocal altruists) collaborating on a vast scale oriented by the social mind and culture that perpetuates it.

For the purpose of this discussion, the Few are defined here as a very small group of individuals. These individuals have acquired control over vast resources of the world through (a) selfish gene/presocial mind motivational attunement, (b) programmed cultural beliefs, assumptions, values, and norms that perpetuate the presocial mind instincts, (c) skill, guile, and sometimes violence, d) entrepreneurship, and in growing numbers, (e) economic inheritance. The idea of a few dominating the world is not just forwarded by some conspiracy theorists. Researchers such as Phillips and Osborne (see *Financial Core of the Transnational Corporate Class*, 2013) have identified a small group of individuals that they claim do just that. According to these researchers, in the world controlled by the West (most of the world), there are some 5,000-7,000 individuals who essentially make all the pivotal decisions for the nations. Of these several thousand individuals between 150-200 of them sit on numerous transnational corporate boards of directors and serve as key hubs of decision making. Although most are from Europe and North America they are comprised of men and women from around the world including Africa, the Middle East, Asia and Latin America. Their views vary on how to manage the proletariat—some prefer Bread and Circus strategies and others the Bible and Bullets approach, for example.

Although the Few are primarily among the proprietors of transnational corporations (members of the billionaire class), they also include totalitarian regimes (e.g., North Korea, China). The distinguishing characteristic of the Few, in addition to the ruthless control of economy, is an absolute commitment to expanding their power and resources, even at the tragic expense of sometimes millions of men, women, and children. The Few are not comprised of only one race, gender, nationality or religion, but have emerged throughout history in all continents across the globe.

Through attributes of the presocial mind, the Few are committed to maintaining and increasing their control of such resources against all challengers. Their power is that they have evolved to represent the most successful manifestation of the presocial mind orientation (selfishness, deceit, and war); they personify the highest achievement of the selfish gene base attributes as conceptualized by Dawkins.

Mutualists (my term) are defined here as those genetically and/or culturally disposed to pursue their goals for society (and cultural evolution) through collaboration because of an innate and/or conscious belief that they are more apt to succeed. Only in large collaborations can they compete with the Few.

The difference between cooperation (such as among oligarchs/ the Few) and authentic collaboration is that cooperation among the Few involves domination by one or more of the participants and a zero-sum orientation. An extreme political expression of this would be corporate totalitarianism or fascism. On the other hand, collaboration is based on equal partnership for equitable outcome. It is a win-win orientation. Its purest political expression is healthy democracy. The *individualists of the ordinary ilk* (non-highly dominant individuals who are zero-sum in their orientation), for the most part would turn out to be a group that is co-opted by the Few, or occasionally involved in collaborations with mutualists (believing no other reasonable option exists). Otherwise the individualist of the ordinary ilk will be relegated to being disempowered marginalized groups or lone wolves.

Individualists of the ordinary ilk would have to cooperate with each other in large numbers in order to compete with the Few and the mutualists. If the individualists of the ordinary ilk successfully developed nonhierarchical cooperatives, they would be well disposed to collaborate with the many, in effect becoming mutualists themselves. If their cooperatives were highly hierarchical, winner-take-all in orientation and extremely successful, they would then be the Few competing with the mutualists. There could be groups that straddle these two extremes, but, overall, what appears is a struggle between the masters of the presocial mind domain in cooperation and the champions of the social mind orientation in collaboration—oligarchy vs. healthy democracy.

What I mean by a healthy democracy is the process of governance of, by, and for all the people in an equitable manner: a reciprocal–altruistic-focused (win-win) government. In order to achieve the common good, the people's work must center on collaboration among equals. Unhealthy democracy is zero-sum focused: a divided government that weakens democracy and makes it susceptible to oligarchic interests and ultimately its demise.

There are dozens of forms of democracy. The *Merriam-Webster* online dictionary defines democracy as "(a) government by the people; *especially*: rule of the majority and (b) a government in which the supreme power is vested in the people and exercised by them directly or indirectly through a system of representation usually involving periodically held free elections." However, *Merriam-Webster* (2017) also noted that, "No consensus exists on how to define democracy, but legal equality, political freedom, and rule of law have been identified as important characteristics. These principles are reflected in all eligible citizens having equal access to legislative process." The dictionary then directed the reader to Waterloo Region District school board, which offered eight generally accepted principles of democracy: (1) personal freedom (religion, speech, etc.); (2) political freedom (right to associate, advocate); (3) political equality (equal access to voting/running for office; (4) rule of law (all subject to the same laws); (5) common good (all have a responsibility to show care toward the common good); (6) human dignity (as a right for all people); (7) being informed and getting involved (a requirement for successful democracy) and (8) respecting others' rights.

According to *Merriam-Webster*, an *oligarchy* is "(1) government by the few; (2) a government in which a small group exercises control especially for corrupt and selfish purposes." Democracy and oligarchy can be present in individual organizations as well as in government.

The battle that has come to a head is the clash between two emerging cultures: the culture of absolute control over the masses imposed by the dominant few for their selfish gain and a culture emerging from the masses looking to mutualism for equitable outcomes. *This is the ongoing battle for the soul of human civilization.* We see this struggle throughout history. It has been marked by brutality, oppression, and guile, but also great heroism and brilliance. We have seen the rise of monarchs, dictators, totalitarians, and robber barons that embody the base instincts that have surfaced during the course of human evolution. Yet in this darkness have emerged glimmers of light—a dim but growing glow of mutualism emerging in response to tyranny. This light pierced through the darkness of ancient Greece, arose from the federalist system of the Iroquois, and broke through the darkness that oppressed the American colonies. It is the light of democracy that serves as a beacon to the world, and the battle for and against it is rooted in our memes and genes.

I submit that the descriptions of Axelrod's Prisoner's Dilemma game experiments (Dawkins 1989; Diamond 2005; Sapolsky, 2005), outlined in this book, can be used to summarize the struggle between healthy democracy and oligarchy that I have described. It is a struggle between cultural evolutionary strategies akin to Tit-for-Tat with forgiveness vs. Defect. Moreover, I propose that like Axelrod's experiment findings, initially, Defect culture prevails, but in the long haul, as long as there is a critical mass of Tit-for-Tat with forgiveness players, the reciprocal-altruistic cultural evolutionary strategy triumphs.

Donald Trump (with his billionaire–Wall Street–militaristic administration) personifies the selfish gene—the presocial mind attributes. He and his ilk are like a class of *Super* Cheats. They are predisposed to avoid reciprocating, particularly to those outside of their families and class. Conversely, healthy democracy encourages the proclivity for reciprocal altruism, through the social mind orientation, to permeate society.

Trump and his ilk's very nature is a dark shadow looming over our psychological, political and social–cultural future, and the nature they personify will use every kind of guile and coercion at its means to crush all rivals—the greatest of which is a healthy democracy.

The 2016 election was not a referendum for or against mutualism. Authentic mutualism was never offered. Both sides claimed to be uniting forces, yet both used identity politics to galvanize a base focused on division. Both sides played the "us against them" meme, but from different perspectives. Both sides were corporatists, and this guaranteed that corporate oligarchy would seize the day. We now have a *corporate* government ("of, for, or belonging to corporations," (*Dictionary.com* 2016), controlled by an oligarchy of billionaires.

According to BBC News, a study by M. Gilens (Princeton University) and B. Page (Northwestern University) has confirmed that the United States is no longer a democracy or a republic.

> Multivariate analysis indicates that economic elites and organized groups representing business interests have substantial independent impacts on US government policy, while average citizens and mass-based interest groups have little or no independent influence.

The assault on mutualism is now on steroids. The election of the Trump–Pence regime has filled many Americans with fear and disdain toward those who voted for them. I struggle with these feelings as well. It's hard for me not to see that, based on the rhetoric and deeds of *some* of the Trump–Pence supporters, these citizens have voted for the oppression of our daughters, the disenfranchisement of millions of Americans, and the threat of violence perpetrated by the likes of the Klan and neo-Nazis. As juxtaposed, as many of the memes that Trump and Pence personify are to democracy, we must also remember, that their supporters, as human beings, are a part of our democracy—they are the co-opted individualists of the ordinary ilk. Many of his supporters were simply deceived. We need as many of them as possible to turn toward mutualism, for their sake as well as ours. We stand against their ideas when they oppose equity with every spark of life we possess, but not their humanity. Instead, we champion authentic mutuality. To forget this is to join Trump and Pence in their assault on the emerging evolution that we, who love democracy, so very much desire.

The 2018 election was only a fledgling's first step towards a healthy democracy. Now the great journey begins. The United States is ground zero for this crossroads of human cultural evolution—it is where democracy's cutting edge collides with Orwell's *1984* high-tech psychological totalitarianism. In the following chapters, I will explore historical aspects as well as the trajectory of this ongoing war between democracy and oligarchy. I will suggest ways wellness and the average man, woman, and child can play a pivotal role in helping to achieve America's greater potential. I will explore how healthy democracy can arise in our daily lives, our organizations, our communities, and our nation.

CHAPTER 2

Genocide and the Corporate Colonization of America

THE INTERESTS OF the super-rich and their industries, particularly the transnational or multinational corporation, have always included control over nations: their resources and populations. According to *Wikipedia* (2012), the first multinational corporation, the Dutch East India Company, was founded in 1602 when the States-General of the Netherlands granted it a twenty-one-year monopoly to carry out colonial activities in Asia. Based on the activities of colonialism then, the impetus for the first transnational corporation was environmental exploitation and profit through the policy and practice of harsh and dehumanizing control over weaker peoples via puppet regimes. This exploitation was achieved through coercion and by dividing the subject populations against themselves.

Colonialism as an expression of imperialism turned the leaders (puppet regimes) of the countries under imperial control against their own people. In exchange for this betrayal, these misleaders received wealth and prestige. They manipulated the masses to turn on each other in order to weaken forces countervailing to imperialistic goals. The process of imperialism that divides humanity against itself in pursuit of power and profit for the Few has metastasized into genocide and war throughout history. The ultimate objective of colonization is to conquer the masses, subjugate them to totalitarianism, and

Handbook for True Democracy

eradicate all hope for human rights, freedom of thought, and authentic democracy.

Colonialism is a term that Americans are familiar with, but few recognize that it is being deployed against them even now, as we speak. The transnational presence of major corporations allows them to function almost as if they are sovereign entities, and they have imposed their influence on the nations of the world through diplomacy or military force via the use of lobbying and media scrutiny that in effect establish puppet regimes. These regimes allow corporations to establish communities loyal to them. The billionaire class and the transnational corporate community that they control are like an imperialistic force. For example, transnational energy corporations (e.g., ExxonMobil in the United States) are now poised to usurp not only the oil in areas of the world where "radical Islam exists" but the natural resources of the United States and elsewhere. Through their political control, they aim to gag and dismantle the government regulatory powers of the United States that could successfully oppose their acquisition of U.S. public lands and mineral rights. The billionaire class has gained control of our resources and media, turned our leaders against us, decimated our democracy, locked us in endless wars for their profit, and are now instigating a new American genocide as cover for their corruption.

The idea of a race war occurring in the United States today, much less one that leads to open genocide, is something that the American people might struggle to see as a real possibility. Yet the United States was born of genocide. The ethnic cleansing of indigenous peoples starting in the Eastern United States, through events such as the Trail of Tears, was a continuation of the mass genocide began by the conquistadores of Spain. Tens of millions of indigenous Americans were victims of the expansion of European civilization across the Americas, including the ethnic cleansing that was the American Indian Wars.

Similarly, the slave trade cost millions of Africans their lives during the Middle Passage. Victims of the Middle Passage were packed like sardines in slave ships for months on end. They died of suffocation,

Genocide and the Corporate Colonization of America

disease, malnutrition, and violence and then were thrown overboard without any modicum of dignity. After the Civil War—in the phase of "freedom and reconstruction," the rise of the Ku Klux Klan initiated a wave of ethnic cleansing. The Klan not only lynched a myriad of black individuals and farmer families, but their ilk, over the following decades, murdered and burned down entire towns made up of African American people. Such events wiped black lives and places off the map of America forever. Others faced ethnic cleansing as well. During the conquest of the Western territories, thousands of Mexicans were brutalized, hung, and chased off lands that their families had lived on for generations. The Chinese also faced lynching and white race riots. In fact, the Chinese and Jews are examples of immigrants who were, at times in our history, barred from entering this country altogether. Moreover, racial aggression of this nature toward communities of color continued well into the twentieth century.

Much of the racially based brutality throughout American history occurred at the hands of white commoners (i.e., not government-sponsored actions). However, the policies that implicitly supported and sometimes explicitly initiated the ethnic cleansing in America almost always emanated from the highest levels of society—the moneyed power elite and the governments that they control.

The genocidal underpinnings of America did not stop with the above obvious examples— it evolved and continues to this day. The Indigenous Americans herded onto reservations and African Americans forced to endure Jim Crow faced such poverty and cultural destruction that the mortality rate and sociocultural deformity for these communities were crushing and continue to reverberate today. The assault on communities of color theoretically evolved from slavery and ethnic cleansing, Indigenous American reservations, and Jim Crow, and then, through the intellectual inspiration of eugenics, to legislation supportive of abortion as a "remedy for poverty." "Family planning" is today emphasized in poor communities of color. Overall society may see these "pro-choice" efforts as benevolent; even so, the result addresses a goal established by the eugenics movement in that it emphasizes the reduction of people of color in America. From this point of view, population control can indeed be described as having an element of ethnic culling—a kinder, gentler form of ethnic cleansing. This matters, because there is political power in numbers.

In the 1980s and 90s, new laws on drug offenses (that implicitly targeted people of color) and the three-strikes laws (even for minor offenses) led to millions of black men and women becoming incarcerated for decades, often for life. This in effect was a powerful birth control imposition that also impeded the growth of the African American community. We cannot confirm that the policies described above were implemented with an eye on ethnic culling. However, the fact that talking about the consequences of these policies is (almost) a social taboo is telling of the implicit aggression that still exists around race in this country. Note the almost violent reaction of some in the media at the very words "Black Lives Matter." It is as if just the notion of lives of black people mattering is, to certain "news" pundits, a threat to white lives. America is steeped in implicit and explicit racial aggression that could lead to full-blown genocide. Full-blown genocide is a part of America's DNA, and it waits, like all DNA, to be activated by the right environment.

The emerging environment for full-blown genocide in America today begins with the will of members of the elite such as Donald Trump and Rupert Murdoch. What (in addition to racial hatred) could motivate such an elite to initiate a campaign of full-blown racial genocide in America today? The answer is this: the same things that motivated the Donald Trumps of American history to commit genocide in the past—a greed and power lust so perverse as to demand control of all resources whatsoever—be it land and slaves or today's prized treasures: Internet, media, crop seeds, even our thoughts and genes. The motivation of the Few for genocide is, and has always been, fear and greed (i.e., the presocial mind). Genocide is a tool used to redirect the anxiety and anger of the masses. It is like a blood sacrifice. It allows the Few to feed their insatiable, narcissistic, psychopathic greed and lust for power while others pay the price for their deeds.

The rise of Trump–Pence represents one group of elites challenging another group for top dog status. Their methods differ but not their goals. If neoliberalism cannot succeed, perhaps a harsher approach will be more expedient. If the likes of the Clintons and Obamas could make tens of millions, even hundreds of millions, of dollars as an indirect result of their presidencies (for themselves, not to mention the billions reaped by their elite sponsors)—what could a man like Trump garner for himself and the Rupert Murdochs of the world? The masses, of course, potentially stand in the way of all these possible acquisitions by the Few. The solution posed by the problem of the masses resisting oppression is and has always been *dividing, conquering, and ruling.*

A prime mechanism for implementing the divide-and-conquer strategy is *us-against-them memes* that blame the victim and thereby establish scapegoats onto whom the Few can deflect their sins. These memes prepare minds to be manipulated into carrying out all kinds of acts on behalf of the Few, including genocide—through war, slavery, or ethnic cleansing.

The minds of those needed to implement the genocide must first be inundated with the emotions of fear, anger, envy, and greed (i.e., the activation of the presocial minds) in order to assimilate the us-against-them memes into their worldview (programmed mind functions/culture) and energize them for activation. The convenient rise of Obama (and the white anger and fear that followed), the success of the black athlete, immigrant workers, Black Lives Matter, Latinos ("fastest growing population in America"), affirmative action, China's economic challenge to America, and, let's not forget, Middle Eastern-inspired terrorism—fill much of white America with all the above emotions. How these images are framed makes all the difference in the world, and they have too often been framed by media coverage in a manner that divides Americans along racial lines. The argument that is used to justify this reporting style is that it's done for ratings. However, it cannot be credibly argued that the media is unaware of the social consequences of this approach.

The act of genocide requires that members of the *in-group* have power over the *out-group*—the group to be exterminated. Initiators of genocide target the defenseless. They target the disabled, the sick, the old, and the poor, the immigrant—the voiceless. The lead target, however, is the defamed, those whom the institutions of the society deem "evil." For example, the popular saying of the nineteenth century, "The only good Indian is a dead Indian" (promoted in the literature of the day) illustrates the tactic, as does the accusation that problems facing post-WWI Germany were the fault of "evil, thieving Jews and Gypsies" (also promoted in the literature of the day).

Genocidal gateway memes (i.e., cultural ideas that open the door to genocide) have continued in America through the decades, e.g., the "superpredator" (black youth) meme that emerged in the 1990s, and today the "rapist, murderous, drug-importing Mexican" (the undocumented Hispanic worker). The idea that terrorism is somehow synonymous with all Muslims and Middle Eastern-looking people is another example. These memes are part of a dehumanization process that grants society permission to harass, oppress, incarcerate, and ultimately target entire groups for murder and ethnic cleansing. Those in-group individuals (e.g., whites) who challenge this system legally, and all that protest it, of course risk being targets as well. In fact, they are the ultimate target, because once the in-group dissenters are subdued, totalitarianism prevails.

The American population has been undergoing a battle for democracy against the Few since it was a colony of the imperial British Empire. The resistance to the Few includes the American Revolution that founded this nation, the Civil War that freed Africans in America from slavery and forged together the Union, the women's right to vote movement that led to the Nineteenth Amendment to the United States Constitution that gave women the right to vote in 1920; the movement to unionize that led to the Wagner Act of 1935 that legitimized collective bargaining, civil rights, and most recently, the gay rights, Tea Party, Occupy, Black Lives Matter, and re-emerging women's rights movements. These awakenings *can* be, of course the greatest threat to the Few who hold economic power over the masses as their core value and prime objective. The Few also can use awakenings of the masses as means to further their desired end. In defense of their power, no guile is too diabolical to employ, including co-opting/instigating social movements and using them like sheep's clothing to conceal their wolf-like predatory intentions. An example of this is the takeover of the Tea Party movement by the billionaire Koch brothers through their financing of its activities and ultimately developing an agenda that further diminishes authentic American democracy.

During the American civil rights movement of the 1950s and 1960s, progressive and religious leaders courageously worked together to continue the transformation of America into a system of all the people, by all the people, and for all the people equitably. But as the Few neutralized the authentic leadership of these movements, the movements began to flounder. Support for these movements was then offered in the form of finances and "organizational development" (legitimacy) from liberal-appearing funding sources (fronts of the Few), but this help came with a price. The conditions were that leaders of these movement organizations would have to be easily co-opted to ensure that the organizations would pursue less radical agendas.

If the political elite had been serious about supporting diversity, they would have developed policies to support the authentic leaders of these movements so that they, along with their communities, could design and develop programs that produce self-determination and empowerment within their communities and our broader democracy. Instead, we saw activist leadership of the 1950s and 1960s (both racial minorities and white) ultimately co-opted (bribed with jobs and high profiles), corrupted (turned against their own causes for the sake of funding), or crushed (delegitimized, defamed, economically destroyed, imprisoned, or killed). Those of their organizations that remained became, for the most part, the fund recipients of the power structure that oppressed them, and their causes often became the tools of the political elite controlled by the Few.

The political elite used many of the remaining organizations associated with these movements of the era as cover for their neoliberal intentions—many of these organizations became surrogates for a Clinton administration whose policies led to the incarceration of millions of people of color that in turn led to the (privatization) prison/slave industrial complex, supported welfare reform that discouraged fathers from being in the homes of their children, and supported trade policy that crushed communities of color and working whites economically. The trend of co-option continues, and both major parties have become the right and left hands of the Few, who now usher in a new colonization through racial and political division: the corporate colonization of America.

In the 1980s, members of the American political and economic elite (driven by the Few) upped their offensive against the progress achieved by many of the above-described awakenings and an emboldened middle class in general. American corporations began to adapt to the challenges posed by unions and civil rights through a new strategy that focused more on the emotional environment of the nation and some of its key human capital. The Few began to focus more on influencing public opinion, elected officials, and legislation. Politicians became a highly valued form of human capital, and corporations began to invest an increasing amount of money and time into developing and nurturing those who pursued corporate goals.

President Ronald Reagan began this new wave of assault on the institutions of our democracy with not only trickle-down economics (an indirect economic assault on the middle class), but also policies that furthered the deregulation of television ownership by increasing the number of stations a single person could own from seven to twelve. In 1985, Reagan abolished limits on television advertising per hour, increasing the influence of big money advertisers on the Fourth Estate. He also eliminated the FCC's Fairness Doctrine that required broadcasters to make every attempt to cover contrasting points of view. President Bill Clinton finished this hit job on the Fourth Estate by signing into law the Telecommunications Act of 1996. This act allowed for an unlimited amount of radio ownership by one person.

Today thirteen companies own the majority of all radio stations, and six companies own almost all the television and cable networks in the United States. The Fourth Estate of our democracy is now squarely in the hands of corporate oligarchy.

The assault on our democracy has been a relay race run by the presidents of our country regardless of what their initial intentions may have been as they entered office. Between 1981 and 1985, the number of lobbyists in Washington essentially quadrupled—dramatically increasing corporate power: In the *Washington Monthly* (2003), *New York Times* political reporter Nicholas Confessore wrote an article entitled "Welcome to the Machine" in which he said, "Savvy GOP operatives steered that money toward the Republican Party." Policy began to tilt further toward industry.

> In August 1981, President Ronald Reagan fired thousands of unionized air traffic controllers for illegally going on strike, an event that marked a turning point in labor relations in America, with lasting repercussions. In the decades before 1981, major work stoppages averaged around 300 per year; today, that number is fewer than thirty (Schalch 2006).

This trend in favor of corporations continued during the era of Clintonomics—the "Third Way" (1990s). The development of policies like NAFTA (North American Free Trade Agreement) weakened unions and led, like never before, to the flow of jobs to cheaper labor markets outside of the United States. With more competition for American jobs, the buying power of the average American continued to decline (Pollin 2000). The deregulation of banking (e.g., the Gramm–Leach–Bliley Act of 1999) during the decade not only allowed Americans to live beyond their means through easy credit opportunities but also put at risk their dwindling savings that could now be affected by Wall Street mismanagement. As a consequence of greater debt, workers became more dependent on their corporate employers and consequently more subservient. Moreover, the economy became increasingly unstable, as did the personal finances of the middle class. The stage was set for the American economic and labor crisis of the early twenty-first century.

Furthermore, during this offensive push to weaken democratic institutions of the United States that began in the 1980s, the CIA's alleged introduction of drugs[2] and illegal guns (that led to gang organizational structure and values) into ghettos became like the new Middle Passage; it brutally transported black youth into (gang culture) activities and ultimately the new Jim Crow and prison industrial-slave complex that followed as a result. The CIA's efforts ultimately worked in concert with the Clinton administration's policies on crime (Violent Crime Control and Law Enforcement Act of 1994) built on the Nixon administration's war on drugs and Reagan's "get tough on crime" memes. But this was just part of the strategy imposed by the Few—globalization and trade agreements created a smaller and smaller piece of the economic pie left for the American masses to fight over (while elites like Trump grew richer).

To manage the growing resentment arising out of trickle-down economics and globalism, there would have to be scapegoats. Right-wing radio talk shows and Fox News worked together to create—through dog-whistle racist reporting and editorials—white anger and fear directed toward blacks, Mexicans, Muslims, and the Chinese. Yet the media has all but ignored the fact that it was the policies of the political and economic elite (the Few) that instigated the above sources of white fear. It was CIA activities, trade agreements, and militaristic foreign policy that led to the rise of ISIS, drug gangs, jobs leaving the United States, and undocumented immigrants entering our country. That was true until very recently, when such information could be twisted to create a new illusion capable of co-opting and galvanizing the white working class (the individualists of the ordinary ilk) against their own interest. That illusion, aka the billionaire populist and master of guile and division Donald Trump, offered America's white working class false hope. Meanwhile, blacks, Hispanics, Muslims,

---

2   See Gary Web's "Dark Alliance" series (1996), *The Mercury News*.

and Chinese have been successfully blamed for white working-class problems and, as far as many white Americans are concerned, should pay the price!

This shifting of responsibility was easily achieved—it played on deeply rooted cultural orientations (programmed beliefs and world views) of the white masses (e.g., fear and rejection of people of color and historic scapegoating of these communities). This practice of scapegoating people of color is an institution of the American media owned by the economic elite. It is the Few who stand to benefit most from racial division because it weakens the working class that they fear could challenge their rule. The more working-class individuals are focused on fighting each other, the less they focus on resisting the dismantling of their democracy.

The election of George W. Bush contributed to the process of corporate oligarchy and dismantling of democratic structure by depleting the treasury through war and monetary policy, gutting the Constitution by ushering in the Patriot Act[3], overstepping of the FISA courts[4], introducing the Military Commissions Act[5], and reinforcing the president's unilateral power as Commander-in-Chief after the events of September 11, 2001. Meanwhile, the billionaire Koch brothers were funding a takeover of local and state governments that led to a gerrymandering tour de force, as well as control of the election process throughout the country by highly corporatist Republican governors bent on voter suppression.

When the piton was passed to Obama, he immediately went to work for the banking industry through banker bailouts, opposing a moratorium on home foreclosures (which damaged the black community) and denying caps on credit card interest, as well as fighting shamelessly for the Trans-Pacific Partnership (TPP) global trade deal.

---

3 Circumvents the I, IV, and VI Amendments of the Constitution.
4 Alleged secret rulings to allow government and corporate identities to secretly spy on citizens not suspected of crimes.
5 Allows government to detain citizens without charge, allows use of evidence obtained by coercion, and allows the president to define torture.

Obama also became the president with the distinction of cracking down on the most whistle-blowers in the history of the United States at the time while simultaneously overseeing the development of the greatest surveillance state in the history of the world. He earned the title of "Deporter in Chief" from many progressive Latino social action organizations in America while expanding military action to Yemen and Africa. He established the precedent of legally killing American citizens while overseas without due process. He also presided over the dismantling of the DFL's fifty-state strategy that won them the presidency and both the Senate and Congress in 2008. With these distinctions, he passed the piton to the Trump–Pence administration with little more than a whimper of resistance, a pat on Trump's back, and a "Good job" to boot. Now Trump is charged with establishing the supremacy of the Executive Branch over the Congress of the United States, thus reducing the legisative branch into a mere corpse of American democracy.

Although each of the above presidents have made important contributions to our nation, (the value of which, of course, is largely determined by one's political orientation), each also, in his own right, has been an agent for the Few. Each of these presidents has offered grand words and grand gestures of reform as a smoke screen for a war on democracy that has now come to a head. The United States two-party political system, along with the media that fan the flames of division, is the primary source for exacerbating the American divide. Moreover, the two-party political system, the centerpiece for this divide-and-conquer strategy, is brilliant, because if we don't participate in it, and the other side wins, we will be punished. So I am not advocating for nonparticipation, but instead, *open-eyed* participation, with a focus on transformation. Both parties must be infiltrated with people committed to empowering the everyday man, woman, and child of this great nation, but from different perspectives—one conservative and the other progressive.

The mask of benevolent globalism (the approach of neoliberalism) worn recently by the political elite driven by the Few has played out. The people oppose trade deals that promote privatization and require society to grant transnational corporations power over local government. Since corporate globalism doesn't sell to the masses, a new mask is now being worn. It is the mask of fascism spun as populism—race and nation over all other values, obscured by the smoke screen of high profile/low substantive jobs initiatives and temporary tariffs designed to steal news headlines, pseudo-trade deals that amount to zero structural change in support of economic democracy and instead more profit for segments of the Few. Since the masses have awakened to the corporate takeover of America from outsiders through trade deals and globalism, the Few now resort to conquest from within through fascism. The result will be the same—the disempowerment of our local governments and our democratic institutions in order for corporate rights to prevail over all.

The *Merriam-Webster* dictionary defines *fascism* as a "regime that exalts nation and often race above the individual and that stands for a centralized autocratic government headed by a dictatorial leader, severe economic and social regimentation, and forcible suppression of the opposition." Trump's authoritarian tendencies along with his "America first" battle cry and reluctance to denounce white nationalism clearly suggest fascism. When we also consider that his stated enemies or problem communities have almost exclusively been communities of color (i.e., the Chinese, the Muslims, Hispanics, "inner city," Iranians, Koreans), whereas those he calls "his people" (i.e., the crowds that attend his rallies that are almost exclusively white) and his friend's (e.g., Russia and other totalitarians), his orientation toward facism is clearly illustrated. When we consider whom he has appointed to run the agencies of the American government, the fascism structure is undeniable. According to David G. Mills (2004),

> The early twentieth century Italians, who invented the word fascism, also had a more descriptive term for the concept— estato corporativo: the corporatist state. Unfortunately for Americans, we have come to equate fascism with its

symptoms, not with its structure. The structure of fascism is corporatism, or the corporate state. The structure of fascism is the union, marriage, merger or fusion of corporate economic power with governmental power. Failing to understand fascism, as the consolidation of corporate economic and governmental power in the hands of a few, is to completely misunderstand what fascism is. It is the consolidation of this power that produces the demagogues and regimes we understand as fascist ones. (1)

Trump took his campaign plays right out of Hitler's playbook. Hitler, using guile, racial animosity, and the "Big Lie," rose to usurp Germen democracy through planting the seeds of genocide that would ultimately be used to crush the unions and still the pulse of German democracy.

The media, in Hitler's time and ours, is the primary apparatus for disseminating the *genocidal gateway* memes that target minorities for scapegoating. Media sources, from *The Economist* (2016) to numerous Fox News sources and *Real Time with Bill Maher,* are calling to normalize "politically incorrect" language and consequently provide the likes of Donald Trump with cover.

It is one thing to oppose the treatment, for example, of a sportscaster who, on one on-air occasion, made a racist comment that resulted in the loss of his entire career. Certainly disciplinary action would be in order; however, such extreme treatment as this can make all of us wrongful victims of political correctness overreach. Such extreme punishments miss the point of political correctness and consequently weaken its standing among the masses. The point of political correctness is to institutionalize the rejection of mainstreaming of language that denigrates an entire people (or group), not to destroy whites that make a one-time slip of the tongue. The mainstreaming of defamatory language lays the psychological foundation for genocide (or misogyny, for that matter), and that's exactly what is happening through this new assault on political correctness. This is happening whether the perpetuators realize it or not.

The cameras of the American genocide consent-manufacturing machine focus their lenses on any little action that supports the notion that the races are a threat to each other. Police brutality illustrates this point. An out-of-control policing system is a general threat to Americans (albeit with a heavy emphasis on people of color). For example, there have been numerous police shootings of unarmed white Americans (e.g., Zach Hammond), but the media, instead of following these cases with the same elevated status as police shootings of racial minorities, buries them. The rare exception, of course, is the shooting of Justine Damond, a forty-year-old Australian white woman who was shot by a Somali American officer in the upper-middle-class neighborhood of Minneapolis, Minnesota where she resided. In this case of course the police officer was convicted of murder. An August 20, 2019 headline for an article written by Gary Joad and Kate Randall underscores this point: "Police Violence the 6th Leading Cause of Death for Young Men in U.S." That's *all young men* between the ages 20 and 35. The article was based on a study published by the Proceedings of the National Academy of Sciences (August 5, 2019). The result is reality is distorted in a manner that encourages racial divide.

Instead of identifying a common problem facing poor and working-class Americans, the media coverage encourages division. Through coverage that suggests that police brutality is a problem facing only the black community, while also instigating fear toward blacks in general, media coverage, in a roundabout way, helps to both pre-justify and minimize future killings of blacks by police.

Since the Few benefit most from racial divide, it is possible that elite entities even purposely help elevate social movements like Black Lives Matter. Police lynching (i.e., police shootings, beatings, or choking to death of unarmed black Americans) has been going on in this country since slavery times. But through the use of the media, awareness of these state-sanctioned killings was elevated just in time to help frame the 2016 election in racial conflict.

The billions of dollars of free media lavished on Donald Trump's suspicious rise not only empowered a figurehead for hate, it served as the gasoline on the fire of the kind of racial conflict needed to turn this country into an open police state! White Nationalism inspired terror is just one avenue that could cause the United States to erupt into all out violence. Under a Trump–Pence administration, the riots or protests against white nationalism could be bloody and the crackdowns brutal. When the conflict spills over into white communities, the stage will be set for the coming race war that of course communities of color cannot possibly win.

Not only do communities of color lack the population, economics, organization, and mass media to defend themselves effectively in a race war, but also preparations supplied by the political policies and programs described above have ensured that such a war would be a slaughter of the bloodiest kind. The CIA-inspired drug (gang) wars (and Clinton policy) not only helped further the political disenfranchisement of black and Latino communities, they helped minimize legal gun ownership in communities of color, while Republican policy encouraged white Americans to legally arm themselves and "stand their ground."

The millions of black felons, for example, often not only lost their right to vote for life, they also lost the right to legally bear arms. The violence in African American and Latino communities created by drug wars (with illegal guns) helped to fuel the Democratic Party mantra for making *legal* purchases of guns more difficult. The antigun meme reproduced itself widely among Democrats, a party of which a very large majority of blacks and Latinos consider themselves to be members. This has resulted in fewer legally armed communities of color. This also means that a smaller percentage of people of color will be legally concealing and carrying during any race war that may emerge. This also means that they will be less trained in using firearms and less able to "stand their ground" legally in the event that they are attacked by Trump followers. Of course, an argument can be made that a black man with a gun is a target for police with or without a permit to carry (e.g., Philando Castile, who was shot to death by a St. Anthony police officer at the same moment he was telling the officer of his legal right to carry). But certainly, the illegal use of guns in self-defense by people of color would summon the full weight of our militarized police apparatus and heavily biased judiciary against these communities.

The antigun lobby became a mainstay cause of the Democratic Party, but it didn't win over the Donald Trump crowd. Instead, it encouraged them to load up on arms and ammunition "before some Democrat could take their guns and ammunition away." More and more white Americans are arming themselves, as encouraged by the NRA and right-wing media groups and personalities like Alex Jones, who have mastered the dog-whistle racist call to arms. Moreover, the message to whites, if one listens carefully to media-celebrated "stand your ground" legal cases—is that in the case of shooting a black man in the name of "self-defense," one will likely not be charged and even less likely to be jailed (e.g., George Zimmerman). Why is this the case? The "superpredator" meme is why.

The implicit consent to shoot down unarmed people of color is even clearer with respect to police killings of unarmed black men and women. In fact, modern-day police lynching of people of color is already becoming normalized in America. We see the killings of unarmed black men and women prominently on the news, and we see that the black community is enraged. We also see time and time again that the police go free (with a couple of extremely rare exceptions, e.g., those occurring conveniently before the 2018 elections). The message is clear, in general—it's perfectly legal for police to kill unarmed blacks. The consequences of this message are twofold. One is retaliation where police are gunned down by unstable shooters who are at best peripherally affiliated with black nationalist groups. This is of course a tragic loss of innocent lives. It also provides the illusion that the black community is a highly militarized threat to white America, justifies further crackdowns on black resistance, and plays perfectly into the hands of white supremacists seeking a race war.

Consequently, knowingly or not, such shooters are agents for the racist elements of Trump's agenda. The other consequence is that nothing changes and whites become one step closer to being accustomed to the "infotainment" news of modern-day lynching of black men and women. Blacks become hopeless. "It is what it is" becomes the norm. Through the media, the lynching of blacks as a community entertainment event becomes institutionalized in American once again.

The difference between a race war and genocide is that a war is a contest between more or less equally armed opponents, whereas in genocide the victim (contrary to propaganda) is essentially unarmed. There can be no race war in America. There can only be ethnic cleansing and full-blown genocide. People of color are no more prepared to defend themselves from an American system bent on their imprisonment and death than the Jews and Gypsies of Nazi Germany were against Hitler.

Trump won the 2016 election and maintained the Senate in 2018. His entire presidency has been a campaign for re-election. He will likely boast the largest re-election campaign war chest in the history of the world and contrive an October surprise of historic proportions. With (essentially) the end of the Voting Rights Act, the purging of voters of color from voter registration lists going largely unchallenged by the Democratic establishment, Republican gerrymandering and Trump's propagandized smoke screen gestures of good will to the black community (more divide and conquer)—are we all but assured the re-election of Trump? His re-election would likely mean racism in America would become legalized once again. With a corporate-sponsored Supreme Court (as well as lower courts) appointed by Trump that confirms the assertion that "racism is pretty much over in America," the removal of the remaining laws protecting communities of color will easily follow. When Trump exercises his "right to change his mind" with respect to his proworker rhetoric and passes antiworker and antisocial safety net laws (because he "got a great deal and your're gonna love it!"), he will have to shift the focus of American workers toward something else and—"it's gonna be big!" When the Trump who has always stabbed American workers in the back shows his true self, (i.e., a man of the Few, by the Few and for the Few), he will have to sacrifice a scapegoat or two to appease the angry masses. In fact, when the American people are betrayed again, after all his rhetoric, he will have to sacrifice a lot of scapegoats, and this is when the race war could come into play.

At this point, the scenario for full-blown genocide could unfold. Through Trump's intimidation of the media (verbally and through law suites, and depending on the composition of the United States legislature, the enactment of laws that allow billionaires to sue media outlets into compliance), little by little, every positive media image of blacks, Latin Americans, Muslims, and others could be replaced by a negative image. There are already virtually no positive images of Middle Easterners in our media today. Under such conditions, violence, possibly false flags, could continue to emerge and serve as justification for further erosion of what little is left of the American Constitution. Moreover, these events could serve as excuses for Gestapo tactics that lead to an overt police state. The drums for war against populations of people of color could begin to beat louder and louder on our news programs—e.g., "the lawless, rogue radical Black Lives Matter" accusations of some "news pundits" (that insinuate that all of these protesters belong in prison or worse) will eventually become simply "Blacks are radical rogues who belong in prison or worse." The so-called mainstream media could come to echo the same sentiments as the right-wing radio talk shows and Fox News, but couch them in a more balanced tone—often echoed by black and brown anchors and reporters. Those journalists who resist would be replaced. With a cowed media, and with the courts, Congress, Senate, and executive branch firmly in Trump's grip, he could take this scenario to the ultimate place of terror.

After new refugees from south of the border have been rounded up and imprisoned or deported, the next phase could be to round up the some eleven million remaining undocumented immigrants from Mexico and Latin America who Trump promised he would deport. Resident aliens, nationalized citizens, and even American soldiers promised citizenship for their service would not be safe. The problems that arise in detaining these immigrants could become the justification to use a "special police force" (also promised by Trump) and "Your papers, please" laws used to harass people of color.

The FEMA housing, really more like concentration camps, that has long awaited use could find justification by detaining these populations. Perhaps other large numbers of people deemed a threat to the elitist Trump who dwells in the White House in the guise of a "populist" could one day find their way to the same fate.

Inspired by apartheid and the occupied territories of the world, the full marginalization (geographically as well as psychologically and politically) of communities of color will have been realized in America when these communities are again overtly segregated through the loss of civil rights in combination with growing business rights that allow discrimination in housing and jobs—even general commerce. Slowly the borders of these segregated communities could be constricted by gentrification after gentrification and skirmish after skirmish (with militarized police) until these communities will be little more than overpopulated detention camps. Whites who oppose Trump–Pence regime policies and stand in solidarity with communities of color would face the full weight of that regime—costing them their livelihood, their freedom, and even their lives. They would be labeled enemy combatants or terrorists, and even their family members would not be safe—a policy enforcement measure that Trump has openly stated that he supports. Gradually the target would grow wider until it includes all of those who openly oppose corporate totalitarianism in America.

As devastating as these events would be for communities of people of color, their primary purpose would be to serve as a distraction, as cover, while the Few pursued their ultimate goal of crushing the white working class. A defeated American population would open the door for usurping all the natural and economic resources of the United States, with an eye on the resources of the world.

In large part, communities of people of color are already under the oppression of the power structure (i.e., economically and politically marginalized, violently oppressed by police, and significantly imprisoned in the industrial/prison/slave complex). The new level of oppression of people of color being offered by the Trump–Pence administration is to provide the white working class with an illusion of elevation (i.e., people that they can look down onto and feel power over). This serves as a distraction while the rights and freedoms of all Americans are being systematically eliminated and their treasury and natural resources ruthlessly plundered. Eventually those of the working class who support Trump will have to face the sobering truth that they too will have to march their children off cliffs—the cliffs of job insecurity, loss of social safety nets, loss of government efforts to address climate change, and the complete destruction of our Constitution and civil liberties.

The crushing of racial (and other) minorities is cover for the final stage of development for a corporate takeover of American democracy that began in earnest many decades earlier. Trump is the latest piece in the plan of corporate totalitarianism that the billionaire class has been orchestrating for over a half century. He quickens the slow, agonizing plunge of their dagger into the heart of democracy, for what the Few have done to people of color overseas, through their political and corporate cohorts, they can now do to communities of color here at home. Whatever they do to communities of color in America foretells of the future of all Americans.

At this writing, of course, in 2020, none of this has occurred under the Trump–Pence administration. But the point is that the deteriorating health of our democracy has led to an environment on the brink of atrocity. If we are honest with ourselves, we must admit that the Trump–Pence rise to power represents a tide of animosity toward diversity, and that horrors such as ethnic cleansing and genocide have historically been built on such sentiments. Animosity toward diversity has been the foundation of genocide and ethnic cleansing not only in other countries, but also in the United States. People in the past have denied the emerging genocide of their day, only to suffer the bitter consequences. Should we do the same now?

CHAPTER 3

The Robber Barons 2.0

THE RISE OF the Few and the economic oligarchy they impose is a new form of colonization. Transnational corporations, corporate conglomerates and totalitarian regimes have in affect acquired political control over the nations of the world and occupy them with local industry that exploits the countries economically. As a result of the success of these oligarchies, it could be said that a form of feudalism is emerging made up of corporate oligarchy vs. corporate oligarchy in competition to control the resources of the world through globalization and military action. The jostling of these economic and militaristic entities for top dog status has led to the most dangerous times in human history. The economic elite of Europe, the United States, Russia, China, and others form pacts constantly threatening one another with guile that could erupt in open conflict at any time. Meanwhile, these pacts suck the life and resources from the nations of the world, exacerbating the gap between the wealthy and lower economic classes and deteriorating the health of humanity and Mother Earth. The government and corporate structures forwarded by the oligarchies of the Few produce inequity and antidemocratic regimes despite promises of populism or benevolent democratic globalism. These circumstances have dire social consequences, as increased power imbalance and oppression could lead the populations of the world toward despair, frustration, scapegoating of minorities, and mass insurrection on a scale never before seen in the history of humankind.

The Robber Barons 2.0

The United States' defacto wars and the potential spread of new wars—both with other nations and with terrorist organizations continue. Militants opposed to domination by the United States (and others they see as the power elites of the world) threaten to retaliate against innocent civilians. These threats, according to media programs such as *60 Minutes*, are magnified by 100 suitcase-sized nuclear weapons unaccounted for from the Russian arsenal. Moreover, tensions over what China sees as its ocean territory could lead to military conflict between the two largest militaries in the world.

As Burke has observed in 2006, the case remains that Russia and the United States have yet to formally step back from their emerging new cold war, and some (e.g., Robert 2007) even suggest a growing threat of World War III. Even with the Strategic Arms Reduction Treaty (START), peace activists such as Lozano (2010) complain "The measure leaves room for the possibilities of new [nuclear] warheads in the future and promises of a big increase in funding for the U.S. nuclear weapons complex." A recent PBS headline illustrates where we are headed: "U.S. Withdrawal of Nuclear Treaty Sparks Arms Race Concerns (August, 2019)." The Trump Administration already has significantly increased the United States military budget. Furthermore, there are several complicating factors. Despite Trump's fawning over Putin, his administration's aggressive stance toward various factions in the Middle East is a potential provocation that could lead to military conflict with Russia, and this could escalate into a nuclear showdown. Moreover, the standoff between the Trump administration and North Korea could ignite a nuclear holocaust, as a war between these nations would likely escalate into a worldwide nuclear conflict.

As if the possibility of a nuclear holocaust were not enough, global warming could end life on Earth, as we now know it. Even more alarming, the Trump–Pence administration's EPA policy appears to indicate that it is not only willing to ignore the science of climate change, but more than willing to accelerate such a future. Not only will global warming displace millions of people, it will result in untold natural disasters, including an astounding loss of species and possible human extinction.

How did we get here? The common denominator for each of the threats described above is major industries run amok. Transnational corporations are the dominant organizations worldwide. Even popular conservatives such as Ron Paul suggest that the financial industry is central to many of the problems facing the United States (see Russo, *America: Freedom to Fascism* 2005). Transnational corporations affect how society is organized, and how society is organized will ultimately determine the destiny of the world. Transnational corporations encourage cash crops instead of crops that feed the hungry. Transnational corporations develop and hard sell, through lobbyists and lawsuits, genetically engineered crops. Transnational corporations also dictate monetary policy in the United States and abroad through Wall Street and the Federal Reserve (a cartel of banks) as well as banking surrogates such as the IMF (International Monetary Fund), the World Bank, and central banking systems the world over. Major industries and their lobbyists encourage not only exorbitant military expenses but also the use of weapons through aggressive militaristic national policy. Furthermore, global warming has been, in large part, attributed to the pollution generated by major corporations that will now be intensified under the Trump administration, particularly those corporations in the energy sector.

The billionaires who control the corporate sector are now openly running the American government. In addition to corporations' influence on policy making throughout the world, they also influence (ultimately, for their own benefit) the world economies through numerous activities, including the control of energy (oil, electricity, natural gas, and coal), the printing of the U.S. dollar, production of food, communications technology, the media, and most major research through partnerships with universities, funding, and media scrutiny (see Greenwald 2012).

Corporations are nonliving entities structurally encouraged to place profit for their shareholders above the environment, their workers, their nations and even the wellbeing of the general public. As long as their actions are technically legal, their bottom line towers over all other goals, as it would be malfeasance for profits not to be the priority. It appears that many major corporations have chosen economic gain over the welfare of humanity. Moreover, they are granted the rights of human beings but with limited liability for their actions. Supreme Court decisions such as Citizens United vs. Federal Election Commission continue to strengthen corporate privilege. The Few, like the anti-Christ of religious lore, have given over their power to the soulless corporate beast. With this legal status and policies such as the Central American Free Trade Act, corporations have gained advantages that supersede the will of our citizenry—they have gained control of the policies, activities, and affairs of our nation—all with limited liability.

In President Eisenhower's farewell address to the nation on January 17, 1961, he expressed concern about the growing power of what he termed the "military-industrial complex." Nearly sixty years later, industry has usurped our democracy. In addition to the re-establishment of a new class of robber barons (corporate dominance) here in the United States, industry has also come to dominate the world.

Contemporary civilization is, in essence, an evolving, extremely complex organization consisting of informal and formal organizations of all sorts, all with varying organizational culture. But the driving organization of civilization today is arguably corporate industry. Industry has become dominant over the governments of the world through its control of information (e.g., television, journalism, and academic research); leadership (e.g., politicians, through political funding); economics (e.g., central banks, IMF, industry); and organization (e.g., control of elections and a legal system that allows for corporations to sue local governments into bankruptcy). In some cases, violent coercion is involved (see Klein 2007). In short, multinational and conglomerate corporations control the pillars of power of contemporary civilization. The pillars of power have come to support the reality imposed on the world by soulless identities—transnational corporations.

The technology used for achieving the goals of the transnational corporation has changed since the establishment of the East Indian Company in 1602, but the goals have not; they are still focused on control of the resources of nations and their populations through puppet regimes and the divide, conquer, and rule strategy. Today this includes the achievement of corporate profits, dominance of markets, and control of consumer, worker, and voter behavior. The pattern of corporate take over of government is consistent—the politicians are lured into establishing huge debt, which in turn is used to justify austerity measures and then privatization is offered as a remedy for the people's pain. The austerity being imposed on Greece is an example of what can happen when governments resist cooperating with the global corporatocracy. The wave of pseudo populism funded by the economic elite that prefers to pursue a more direct approach to usurping the democracies of the world through neofascism is an example of what the oligarchy offers when the people begin to successfully reject globalism. In either case, democracy is compromised. Consequently, these corporations are collectively more influential than any current nation and possess more widespread influence than any past empire.

In the first two decades of the twenty-first century, humanity entered an age of astounding technological advancement. Computer–brain interfacing took the first steps toward reading the human mind. Scientists identified the mechanism for creating invisibility. Super surveillance equipment emerged that is capable of monitoring every telephone conversation in the United States. The technology to track and intimately monitor every human being on Earth is no longer the domain of science fiction but an emerging reality.

History suggests that not only is it likely that industry will use whatever technology is available to achieve its goals, but also that workers (if possible) will quickly adapt themselves to these emerging technologies in order to retain a place in the corporate social order. The greater the role that industry has in society, the more weight workers will place on conforming to the goals of their employers—especially as jobs grow scarcer due to advancing technology and enhanced corporate rights.

The technology used by workers in the past to adapt to the requirements of industry has been acquisition of skills with manual tools of the trades, the ability to use machinery, higher education, and more recently, skills in utilizing high-tech applications. However, more and more, industry requires workers to be innately disposed, both psychologically and genetically, to help further the goals of the employer. For example, since one of the costliest items facing industry has been health care insurance, efforts have been made to require genetic testing of employees for predisposition to illnesses such as lung disease. Disease emerging from such a predisposition could later be blamed on the work environment and result in insurance compensation for the worker. Such claims could affect the cost of employer premiums. In a U.S. News and World Report article published in 2002, Thomas Hayden describes how scientists have successfully manipulated the genetics of fruit flies:

> Now "evo-devo" biologists, who study how fertilized egg cells develop into adults, are discovering powerful new ways evolution can transform organisms. They are finding that changes in a handful of key genes that control development can be enough to drastically reshape an animal.

Moreover, some scientists already claim to have discovered the "violent gene" (i.e., HTR2B) in Finnish men and have been able to turn its analog in rats off and on (Firth, 2012). Could the "questioning-authority-gene" or the "I-don't-believe-in-work-benefits gene" one day be discovered? Could turning off or on such genes become an employment prerequisite? Such possibilities may not be far off. Using genetic tweaking, scientists are already manipulating reality by creating false memories. Perry (2017) noted, "MIT researchers Steve Ramirez and Xu Liu recently made history when they successfully implanted a false memory into the mind of a mouse (1)."

Articles by Cha (2017) in the *Washington Post* with the title

"First Human Editing Experiment in U.S. 'Corrects' Gene for Heart Condition" and "Chinese Scientists who Edited Genes of Twin Girls May Have Supercharged Their Brains" by Rahhal (2019) illustrates how quickly these possibilities are becoming reality. More telling is Kat Eschner's (2018) Popular Science article "CRISPR Has Many Promising Applications—But The Gene-Edited Twins Represent Something More Troubling,' suggest that Chinese Scientists have already successfully edited the genes of living humans that could be passed on to future generations. As technology evolves and our ability to map and understand our genetic codes increases, the potential for employers to demand genetic knowledge about workers as a precondition to employment is very likely to increase as well.

One of the greatest challenges to the goals of industry is its workforce: managing worker behavior and employee demands on the organization economically. Industry is structured to maximize profit at all costs, as long as what they do is technically legal. Why wouldn't industry, particularly in a highly competitive job market, seek out those who could demonstrate—by choice—a genetic predisposition that would best meet the requirements of industry? If altered memories would produce happier employees even under horrific working conditions, why not encourage it? And if the job market were competitive enough, and corporate rights over workers strong enough, wouldn't it be tempting for some to genetically alter their offspring-to-be in order for their children to be more desirable to the corporate world? In fact, wouldn't some parents be willing to genetically "design" their children in order for them to have a better chance at surviving and flourishing as corporate employees?

We are no longer talking about merely changing the eye color or even gender of the child (which some parents are already doing), but potentially changing the gene pool. The idea of technology capable of altering genes that could be passed on is the essence of biological evolution. Could our children evolve into a subspecies of humanity genetically designed to serve corporate goals? Who would these children belong to? Since corporations have the rights of people, don't they have a right to procreate? Corporations will own the patents to these altered genes. So does this mean our children and their offspring could become commodities like other genetically modified organisms (GMOs)? Will our children become the property of the transnational corporations of the world?

History reveals that the nature of workers challenges the goals of industry. It is also clear that industry is committed to using emerging technologies to efficiently focus the behavior of workers toward corporate goals. Are we destined to enter an era of a *genetic man theory*, an era by which organization occurs, not only through the manipulation of structure, group dynamics, psychological conditioning, or other environmental factors, but also through genetic manipulation? Could the proprietors of corporate totalitarianism rise to be the sovereigns of such darkness worldwide? Will a more democratically driven adaptation, like unionism against the industrialists of the nineteenth and early twentieth centuries, emerge today in response to the new technologies of oppression? Could an adaptation to growing corporate domination already be occurring—one where the masses have more self-determination? The following chapters will be an exploration of some proposed answers to these daunting questions.

CHAPTER 4

The Myth of the All-Powerful Corporate Oligarchy

TODAY, MANY OF us find ourselves paralyzed with fear when we think of world developments. The rise of the Trump–Pence reality is like a nightmare that has come to real life. The American police state haunts our streets. Many of us believe that we have an economy built on quicksand and at any moment we could be sucked into the abyss. With the further deregulation of banking, as pursued by the Trump–Pence administration, even our savings accounts may not be safe when our economy fails. The Few and those who cooperate with them control our government through a system of legalized bribery, voter disenfranchisement, and media complicity. To our terror, this unholy alliance is quickly dismantling our civil, constitutional, and human rights. Climate change and all its perils, wars, and the drive toward continuous war, possibly a World War III, loom over the future of humanity.

These terrors infiltrate every aspect of our lives and seem to have us surrounded. We can sense the beast behind these developments everywhere we look: in our watersheds, at work, at the movies, at our banks, at the cameras pointing at us as we drive down the street. It tracks our every purchase and every search we make on the Internet, compiling our psychological profiles in order to predict our future behavior. The system that drives the darkness that threatens our way

The Myth of the All-Powerful Corporate Oligarchy

of life and our future seems omnipresent, omnipotent, and with the rise of super technology and the surveillance state—omniscient.

It is almost as if a powerful anti-Christ has risen from the greed and the technological and economic apparatus that has emerged out of imperialism, the industrial revolution, and modern-day espionage and warfare. Entire nation-states crumble before this power—what chance do the average man, woman, and child have against such a Goliath?

Throughout history, and currently throughout the world, we can see brilliant and heroic men, women, and children making great stands against those who would perpetuate devastating developments against humanity and nature. These are exceptional individuals lifted by exceptional moments in time to do exceptional things, but what about the rest of us who feel a desire to contribute in a meaningful and powerful way? How can we be better, more exceptional in our everyday lives? How can we better ourselves in order to better the world?

Ironically, the response to the ominous dark shadow that hovers over our civilization is found in the lives and behaviors of common folk—we, the everyday men, women, and children of the world. In fact, only we can turn the tide. The Few and those who cooperate with them have galvanized the largest force ever assembled in an assault against democracy and the middle and lower economic classes of the world. In the past, successful peaceful (and not so peaceful) efforts to challenge economic-based injustice arose in waves of large numbers of souls exerting their will to topple oppressive elements. The movement for unionism in the earlier part of the twentieth century and the nonviolent movements that lifted the goals of Gandhi and Martin Luther King, Jr. to fruition are examples. But the Few and those who cooperate with them are well aware of this trend and now have positioned their apparatus to shape media coverage that supports their cause while downgrading the causes of the many.

In the past, the mainstream press at times spread the messages of progressive movements to the benefit of those movements. Today the

49

Few and those who cooperate with them manage the press and are able to use the media to spread misinformation, division, and diversion. The Few and those who cooperate with them now overwhelm these movements' resources with counter-resources and counter-movements; they infiltrate, confuse, and divide movement organizations. The Few are now better able than ever to buy off, discredit, imprison, or kill the leadership of these mass movements with legal impunity and media cover. With these developments, what are we left with? What do we have that can stand against this great force that scatters our numbers? The answer is *you*, and through you—the answer is still—*us*. When we are scattered, we become seeds in the wind. We become seeds of change! Seeds are powerful forces that change landscapes, seemingly overnight.

What force is large enough to topple the oppression imposed by the Few and their alliances? The answer is found in our collective individual actions. You are tiny in comparison to the apparatus of the economic and political oligarchy—but you are a force. You cannot save the world. Only the world can save the world. But you are part of the world, and you can do your part.

Through the way you and a critical mass of other men, women, and children live their lives, the power to topple the seemingly invincible forces of the Few exists. Through personal commitment to wellness and a sense of social responsibility in how we live, we can contribute to loosening the stranglehold that the Few and their alliances have over our democracy. Our focus is not to control others; our focus is to do our part, and that is to control our own lives. Our focus is then to direct our own actions down a path that does not comply with the self-destructive behaviors encouraged by those who would oppress us, and we will passively resist the corporate oligarchy that is the apparatus of the ruling class. Granted, this will take others doing the same, but our task is to do *what we can do* to be healthier and contribute to a healthier democracy.

What we can do is work on ourselves, and work on our actions. There *is* hope, and *you* are it. We as individuals can make choices

The Myth of the All-Powerful Corporate Oligarchy

daily that impact the world in small ways and save our bodies, minds, and souls in the process.

I'm not here to discourage progressive organizing of protests, grassroots lobbying, or civil disobedience—on the contrary! All those things start with individuals' choices of action. Many things will have to occur and contribute to the fall of corporate oligarchy. But I'm here to say that none is more important than what you do to save your life and that of your family and your community. You don't have to be a superhero to achieve this—you just have to make up your mind that change *is going to happen*—at least in how you live *your* life.

Webopedia.yourdictionary.com defines *passive resistance* as "noncooperation or noncompliance with the laws or directives of an authority, particularly of a government or occupying power [e.g., the corporate oligarchs], as a form of protest against injustice." What is proposed in this book is not so much a protest against government as it is against the occupying powers that have imposed their will on *our* democracy and the implicit directives put forth by a system of consumerism that has poisoned not only our environment, but also our bodies, minds, and souls.

Through holistic practices, we can wean ourselves off the physical, psychological, and spiritual toxins that affect our will and our capacity to contribute at least one free, happy, and healthy individual to the world. And by doing so, we can help create a chain reaction that forms a critical mass of behavior that changes the direction of society. For example, as more of us demand organic foods, more and more food producers will grow organically to profit by catering to our requirements. As a consequence, less chemicals and GMOs will be dumped into our environment. The action of demanding more organic foods is one form of passive resistance in order to achieve a more just food supply, because it requires noncooperation with authorities that state GMOs and pesticides are safe for human consumption (and our environment). These actions also create new economic forces that can serve as a countervailing force against the big lobby that encourages GMOs and pesticide use.

The countervailing economic forces alluded to here offer the potential to influence politicians and consequently the development of policies and laws that better address our need for healthier foods and environment. This chain reaction further results in a cleaner environment and a reduced influence of the Few and the destructive effect of their alliances on our civilization. This change started when the first organic farmer offered an organic product for sale and the first customer picked up an organic product and chose it instead of pesticide-ridden or GMO produce. I'm not talking about boycotts, I'm talking about creating a new way of life that zeroes in on the kind of businesses that exhibit the values that you want to see replicated in the world. I'm talking about the first pillar of power—control of economics. We must be the Grudgers (described by Dawkins in his seminal work *The Selfish Gene*), and when we see industry infringing on our health or healthy democracy, we must cease to groom them!

We, the everyday people of the United States, have a long history of boycotts. But what I'm talking about is creating and promoting a new consumer culture that is deeply committed to social change—a healthier, cleaner, and more equitable world. Question the business ethics of those you purchase your goods from, as well as the messages their products promote. Be selective in where you invest your money. Encourage the business where you work to follow suit, if feasible. Lobby your local government to do the same. Keep your ear to the ground with stores where you shop with respect to their employee practices, tax avoidance, environmental records, and the politicians they fund as well as what policies those politicians support!

Sometimes this is as easy as Googling (I suggest using Ecosia.com) the question or asking Siri on your smartphone. Start with the companies that you support regularly: your bank (is it a credit union, community bank, or transnational corporate bank), the insurance company and hospital you use (nonprofit or for-profit organization), the clothes you wear, the movies you watch, the music you purchase, and the car you drive. Be committed. It may not always be possible to buy from a preferred vendor, but it is possible to look for every

The Myth of the All-Powerful Corporate Oligarchy

opportunity to do so, and take every opportunity that presents itself. Be open with others about the reason you use to make your purchases and why that is important—especially those individuals you may have influence over, such as friends and family. Be your own vendor by purchasing organic heirloom seeds and growing a garden. Perhaps instead you can join a community/cooperative garden or grocery store—these efforts can help promote food sovereignty. Support other types of cooperatives or start your own, if you are up to the task. Sometimes your efforts may be more time consuming or more expensive, sometimes product choice as a result may not be exactly what you are used to, but it will be true to yourself and thousands, even millions, of others who feel as you do.

What I'm talking about is changing the economy one consumer at a time. After all, that is how this economy was built—one consumer at a time! Control of economics is a pillar of power. Erect this pillar in your life as a step toward economic freedom for yourself—and the many.

Our choices as consumers affect our reality and the reality of others because we are all connected. Becoming aware of the ripples that emanate from our individual actions into society is the first step in consciously initiating healing actions as a strategy for change. Like the proverbial tossed pebble causes ripples in the pond, we cause small ripples of change in society when we act according to our conscience. Consciously pursuing such change is an act of social responsibility.

Wikipedia.com describes *social responsibility* as "an ethical ideology or theory that an entity, be it an organization or individual, has an obligation to act to benefit society at large." Through social responsibility and passive resistance, we connect ourselves to a large and leaderless, decentralized movement for change that exists throughout the world. Make no mistake—you are not the only one that is awakening. We are in the dawn of world change, and the change that is happening is you!

CHAPTER 5

Out of Darkness Comes Light

MY JOURNEY ON the path to holistic health and social responsibility covers more than a half century. It comprises a patchwork of starts and stops—stumbles, failures, and experimentations with diverse wellness approaches and commitment to social change work. This journey has led me to realize the many profound connections, not only among wellness approaches, but also between wellness and social change. These realizations have been personally transformative. I don't consider myself a foremost authority on meditation and yoga or a master of martial arts energy work. I'm not a food and fitness guru or a renowned healer in an ancient Asian tradition. I'm not a celebrated psychologist. I am an average man, a deeply flawed individual, in fact (like most, if not all, of us). I am on a journey of continuous improvement through using systems that release peace and *agape* (unconditional, altruistic love) into the mind, body, and soul. As a retired man now in my senior years, I have lived a productive, happy, and (for the most part) healthy life against the odds. And against the odds, I have become committed to a better self, and through self-reform, I have been able to help, in small ways, create a better world in which to live.

I was born to a single teenager at the forefront of the wave of fatherless children in America in the decades following WWII. We lived in a small home shared by her five younger brothers, her mother, and her mother's partly live-in boyfriend (mostly on the weekends because he was active in the Air Force). My five uncles and I shared three mattresses located on the floor of our unheated attic-turned-bedroom during the snowy, subzero winters and smoldering summer nights of my youth. My mother and grandmother (thanks to welfare) had their own rooms on the first floor with heat.

I am the fourth consecutive generation born into broken and dysfunctional family life. Abuse disfigured the very image and meaning of healthy relationships in my eyes as I grew up. Witnessing beatings, stabbings, and shootings in the home and on our front doorstep was pabulum for my growing mind. Crime came naturally. Outside of the mainstream where I stood, all parts of the established system seemed to warrant contempt. Deeply embedded in the despair of the lowest economic tier of the United States, I was told time and again that I was destined for prison and probably an early grave. After all, that is how life appeared to end for most of us in my world, so at the time, it was a logical projection.

I remember my childhood with amazing clarity. Although I am a man of average short-term memory at best, I have an astounding memory of my very, very early childhood. Among these memories is me in yellow-and-white onesie pajamas navigating under the table in our dining room, deeply engrossed in the thrill of mastering crawling. I remember standing and walking for the first time. I was alone in our living room sitting on the wood floor across from our sofa (the sofa was green with a kind of towel-like upholstery). It was like a peak athletic experience to stand and stumble forward to that sofa.

I also have dark memories of being filled with blind, violent rage. I remember temper tantrums so severe that I would lose my breath kicking and screaming on the floor until adults scrambled over with concern that I would pass out—or ignored me until I did. It would be easy to blame this rage entirely on my environment. It did play a role (a series of concussions as a youth may have contributed), but violent rage reared its ferocious face at such an early age in my life that I always believed that my condition is partly innate. Ironically, it was this violent rage that launched my journey into the alternative self-realization practices I have been talking about.

My mother and grandmother didn't get along well. My mother moved out of my grandmother's home when I was a toddler, leaving my grandmother to raise me. I couldn't have been much more than one year old at the time, but I remember longing for my mother—waiting for her to return. She never did. So, at six years of age, I decided to return to her.

My grandmother had always been very protective of me when it came to my uncles. My uncles were a close-knit group with much love between them. Nonetheless, they were rough and tumble and sometimes could be horribly abusive to each other and to me. Eventually, my grandmother began working full time and returned to school to get her associates' degree, leaving me in my uncles' care. Without my grandmother's protection, they took every opportunity to let me know where I was in the pecking order. One late summer night, at age six, fed up with their abuse, I hit the city streets and eventually found my way to my mother's home some miles away. It was decided I would be allowed to stay with my mother.

My mother's life was a mess. There was violence in and around our home. Drugs and every type of crime that one could imagine reared their ugly heads in and about my world. But a fundamental shift was about to take place in our lives—that shift was wellness.

Immediately upon entering school, I had begun to act out. Unprovoked violence and disruption emanated from deep within my very being, and everywhere I went, chaos followed. Eventually, after sending me home for fighting (a common occurrence), the school told my mother that they wanted me to be evaluated psychologically or I wouldn't be allowed back.

I was sent to a psychological institution for evaluation. I believe I stayed there for about a week. I was deemed "hyperactive," according to my mother, and the doctors at the institution wanted to put me on drugs. My mother, who had recently been strung out on barbiturates, but kicked the habit by camping out on our couch for a couple weeks in her robe, panicked at the thought of me being on drugs. She stumbled across something called *meditation* and decided to introduce the practice to me instead. I was about seven years old at the time.

Something shifted in me as I meditated. I still had a violent temper, but it was intermittent. In time, violence was no longer a constant, day-to-day, moment-to-moment occurrence. At this time, I was also experiencing joint pain and other health symptoms. Although doctors could find inflammation, they never really were able to offer a firm diagnosis. My mother's response was to begin experimenting with alternative diets and wellness practices. We explored veganism and lactose vegetarianism. We studied yoga and also macrobiotics, eventually moving to Boston to study with Michio Kushi, one of the founders of that movement. We practiced *do-in*, (a combination of breathing and energy exercises and self-massage) and studied various Eastern philosophies and numerous other esoteric and wellness approaches. I was just a little boy, but as my mother's only sounding board, I was filled by her with these new age teachings and practices that had begun to spread in the 1960s. Most of these impacted my health and well-being for the better.

I must have been nine or ten when I first felt the connection that I call our "greater essence." I was outside raking leaves when the feeling overwhelmed me. It made me feel vast, peaceful, joyful, and somehow profoundly drawn to simplicity.

I continued this journey as an adult, involving myself in numerous other studies such as anger management, martial arts energy work, positive thinking and visualization, Transcendental Meditation, and herbal and vitamin supplements. I was like the proverbial monkey going from tree to tree tasting various fruits. There were also periods when my focus on wellness incrementally fell away. I smoked cigarettes, binge-drank, and like many youths, experimented with various illicit substances. The violence and joint inflammation and other symptoms would then re-emerge, little by little, until I refocused on wellness, often inspired by a new practice or philosophy that I had come across.

I wish that I could tell you that I have found the answers to all my problems, but that would be a lie. I never found perfection, and I believe I never will, not in this life. It is likely that I will always work to manage my anger. Even as I write this book, I have struggled with transcending anger during periods of prolonged stress and fatigue. As long as I stay away from certain foods, exercise and meditate I seem to do fine. My anger has become much less severe and is no longer violent, but it is still a part of who I am. But what I can say is that my anger is no longer preventing me from having constructive professional and loving personal relationships. Managing my anger through these practices has allowed me enough of a footing to live a constructive life. Against all odds, I have found a happy and, overall, a very healthy lifestyle—a wonderful family that I love more than anything, a successful career, and occasions to contribute in meaningful ways to bettering my community. It has been a long way to come from the darkness that I was born into, and it is my intent to journey the long way yet to go toward my healing.

As my life progressed, my consciousness expanded and my social awareness blossomed. I began involving myself in social change organizations. Much of this work was about bringing together diversity in order to pursue happier, healthier, and more peaceful and effective organizations and communities. I began to formally study psychology (behavior science, organizational behavior, and organizational development) and eventually earned a doctorate. What I realized was that the healing of organizations, and ultimately society is really about healing relationships, and this begins with healing ourselves. This healing helps us to better pursue caring for others, and it facilitates our contributions to society. Healing the organization is about helping the members improve, and increasing their capacity to create productive relationships in order to pursue common goals. It is about helping participants cooperatively put their gifts to work for something greater than themselves to achieve mutual satisfaction. Involving myself in this change at a personal and professional level was a part of a continuum for my personal growth.

Slowly, over time, I began to combine various practices and wellness approaches that seemed to work for me as learned through my years of trial and experimentation. I found a growing sense of balance to my being, clarity to my thinking, and organization to my life, and this has shaped how I participate in the process of organization and society in general.

As the years passed, I not only managed to build a constructive life, I also began to see through the fog of the debilitating general and early socialization that had clouded my consciousness emotionally, intellectually, and spiritually—releasing into my life not only a greater sense of peace, but also freedom from a form of serfdom that had become more and more apparent to me. I began to nourish the systems of my mind, my body, and my soul. I began to grow into a freer, more independent, healthier human being.

In our journey through life, deep in the soul of each of us there is a drive to realize an ideal state of being. We spend our lives wandering paths with hopes and expectations that they will lead us to reaching this ideal state of life. Sometimes we seek this state in drugs, sex, or other people's approval. We strive for money, recognition, and sometimes redemption; we go to church; perhaps we meditate or fight for political causes. These various endeavors can help us toward achieving this goal, yet something remains amiss. We find ourselves caught up in diversion after diversion, leaving still unmanifested what we sense is our ideal state of being. Why?

Something or some things are not quite in order. Perhaps we sense our political and economic systems are leading us into a destructive way of life. Maybe it's physical—we feel a lack of energy or a nagging pain in our body, and this clouds our vision of a better state of being. Sometimes it's a feeling of sadness or a sense that we are not loved and we are all alone that obscures our view of a better existence. Sometimes we are not sure what is lacking. We know something is out of balance because we sense that we are falling—and helplessness in righting ourselves pursues our souls. Where is our balance?

Balance is characterized in numerous ways, such as "mental

steadiness or emotional stability; habit of calm behavior, judgment; to adjust a chemical equation [perhaps in our bodies]; a symbol of justice; the power to influence or control" (*Dictionary.com* 2018). We are seeking balance in our physical structures—organs, skeletal, muscular, chemical, and neurological—as well as for our emotions, rational mind, and subtle energies.

If we could find authentic balance in our lives, perhaps we could regain our footing as we stumble along our journey, gaining more control and clarity along the way. But to have balance, we must find our center. To find our center, we must know what we are and what we are not. We must understand that all things, including our purest state of being, manifest in the physical world through *systems*. We are all made up of systems because we are made of interacting, interrelated, and interdependent elements. These systems can produce health and harmony, but when malfunctioning, they perpetuate disease and destruction. To achieve healthy systems, we are all compelled to interact with our environments on a continuous basis: we breathe, we consume food and water, we interact with others, and we participate in society—all as matters of survival. This need to constantly interact with our environment means that the human organism is an open system. Environments have an impact on open systems, but this can be mutual. Open systems can establish mutual dependencies with the environment they interact with, causing them to evolve to the benefit of the open system. Balancing the elements within us, and balancing our lives in relation to our environment, is at the center of what it is to be a healthy human being and to participate in a healthy democracy.

CHAPTER 6

Centering the Conscious Mind

There is only one truth, but our minds fragment it into countless pieces that we then exalt separately out of context as the one complete truth.

FOR THOUSANDS OF years, our sages and spiritual leaders have suggested that we are all one and therefore our brother's keeper. Ironically, our physicists have concluded that we, at our most fundamental level, are made entirely of energy. Every material thing—electron, molecule, and cell; every light particle, form of motion, and range of temperature; every emotion and thought—all things in existence are energy, and all energy is connected. Indeed, we are not separate; we are one. Perhaps some energy resonates at a lower level or is denser than other energy—forming different manifestations (physical forms, spiritual dimensions—measurable and nonmeasurable existence), which nonetheless remain connected. Treating our neighbor as ourselves makes sense because they are what we are. We are inseparable in the deepest sense, because our greater essence is energy, and all energy is connected.

Some quantum physicists challenge classical physics altogether by suggesting that, outside of pure energy, there may not be deep reality at all. Even electrons may not have definite existence before measurement. In his book *Quantum Reality* (1987, 159), Nick Herbert noted that some leading physicists have come to "believe that when an electron is not being measured, it has no definite dynamic attributes." According to Herbert (1987, 113-114),

> Some physicists would like to blame the quantum dilemma on the observer's inevitable disturbance of what he measures. However, if we take quantum theory seriously as a picture of what's really going on, each measurement does more than disturb: it profoundly reshapes the very fabric of reality.

What does this mean? It suggests, among other things, that reality, as we conceive it, follows consciousness. It means that fundamental material elements seem to appear and disappear depending on our focus of consciousness—and that reality is, in a sense, the construct of the human mind—which in turn suggests that at the deepest level, energy follows consciousness. The idea, even metaphorically, that energy follows consciousness and that this creates reality has great practical significance for our lives.

Perhaps the source of all being acts as a *possibility wave* (as described by quantum physicists), and the democracy of our interacting consciousness is what forms reality—at least *our* reality. If we collectively choose reality, we then theoretically choose the type of world we live in (Promised Land, Armageddon, and everything in between).

Maybe what physicists call a *lack of deep reality* (i.e., the inability to truly measure the fundamental fabric of the universe) really refers to the oneness of all things in perfect harmony before the mind differentiates them—before the mind shatters the oneness into countless pieces small enough to grasp.

Through our greater essence, we are all connected and therefore are a part of all things knowable and unknowable. The deeper we focus on the connection of all things, the more we can see oneness and harmony in all things. If we could view our greater essence in its unimaginable immenseness, we could envision perfect balance, complete harmony, and perfect peace. So perfect could the balance, harmony, and peace be that it would be outside of existence, as we know it: outside of deep reality. It would be nothingness, because it would be outside of time and space—even outside of change. But from this nothingness comes all things. Hence the Taoist saying: "All things and nothing."

The problem may be that whenever we focus our consciousness on something—from our mother-in-law to the Milky Way—we can't see it in the full context of all existence. Consequently, this out-of-context view is always of an imbalanced nature. So in this sense, all physical manifestations are imbalanced due to the limited ability of human consciousness to place them in the full context of existence. In the context of human consciousness, nothing is perfectly balanced, and therefore all things are made of at least somewhat nonstatic energy—that is, imbalanced reality, or matter seeking greater balance, as water seeks equilibrium. That is why all things appear to change; all things cycle in and out of existence. But not all things are equally imbalanced. Some things are greatly balanced, comparatively speaking, while other things are greatly imbalanced.

There *is* deep reality, and it is from whence all things come—complete oneness and perfect harmony—the connected-energy-of-all-existence—nothingness. But to the extent that this is possible, what does it mean to have this deep reality manifested in our consciousness? It means a greater sense of oneness. It means realizing the connection of all things. It means peace. It means harmony. It means love.

All things are manifestations of our greater essence. Our greater essence is manifest in what we frame as the physical world through systems of materialization. These systems include multiple universes, solar systems, cellular systems, nervous systems, ecosystems, cognitive systems, and even the systems created by the mind, such as organizations, political institutions, and economies. To center the systems created by the mind, we must center the mind on our greater essence. But to achieve this, we must first understand that the mind is a system of the self, and our greater essence is ultimately selfless.

It is helpful to consider the idea that there are two core values from which all values and ultimately human behavior flow:

1) the value of our greater essence (as previously outlined)
2) the value of the self.

These values are of course connected and are not mutually exclusive. However, they do represent different focuses and consequently manifest different realities here on Earth, because energy follows consciousness.

The value of the self is nicely summed up in the attributes of the selfish gene, as described by Richard Dawkins (1989). Dawkins described humans as essentially biological mechanisms that have evolved to perpetuate genes and memes (cultural ideas)—namely, their own. Also, according to Dawkins, we are in a sense programmed by our genes and memes to see those not closely related to us as part of the environment and that either get in the way of our prime objective (the wants and needs of the individual self) or as something to be utilized for selfish purposes.

To some degree, all of us construct our worldview on the value of the self. Most of us include extensions of ourselves such as family, friends, race, and groups (political, religious, and national). In fact, at times we can be quite unselfish in defense of these extensions of ourselves. Extensions of us can also include material objects. However, material objects are obviously not human, and the more we identify with them, the more we dehumanize ourselves and therefore alienate ourselves from the humanity of others. Perhaps that is why research suggests that the wealthy are less empathetic than the poor (Kraus and Piff 2011).

As we entrench ourselves into these constructed realities, based primarily on the value of the self, we begin to lose touch with our deeper identity—our greater essence, or energy (our connection to all things). Eventually, our worldview becomes based solely on the value of the self, and we *become* our worldview, in our mind. We defend our worldview as if it *were* our very essence. That is why we are willing to sometimes harm, even kill, those who severely threaten our worldview. Our worldviews construct our realities. Energy follows consciousness. The lens provided by our worldview can direct energy to construct imbalanced systems in our minds and bodies as well as our environment—including our organizations, governments, economic systems, and religious institutions.

A balanced worldview is a consciousness built on both the value of our greater essence and the value of the self. Our greater essence is inclusive and provides awareness of our connections despite divergent worldviews based solely on the value of the self. It brings balance because it informs us that what we *really* are cannot be threatened by divergent worldviews, because they are a part of what we are. We are energy, and in the deepest sense, energy cannot be destroyed. We also realize, as Chief Seattle explained so eloquently, "Whatever befalls the Earth, befalls the sons and daughters of the Earth."

As individuals, we are all born unique, and we cannot be other than who we are. However, we can focus our consciousness on our greater essence and achieve a more balanced version of ourselves. Each of us is born uniquely oriented to the world—with our own dispositions and inclinations, strengths and weaknesses. Some of us tend to be pessimistic and others hopeful. Some of us are born with easily damaged knees and others are born with exceptional overall physical strength. We cannot completely change our nature as set forth at birth, but we can diminish or optimize our potential. For example, we may be genetically predisposed to cancer, but we can be extra vigilant in avoiding conditions of the mind, heart, body, and environment that trigger cancer—perhaps forestalling it or even avoiding it all together. Conversely, perhaps we were born with a rock-solid physical constitution, but through drug abuse, we have prematurely crashed the systems of our body.

Our worldviews shape our cultures. Our lives reflect our cultural identities. This means that, based on beliefs and assumptions about the world and our values, we generate norms of behavior. Cultural artifacts such as social symbols, sacred texts or relics, credos (e.g., the

Constitution of the United States), and other symbols support these norms and values, beliefs and assumptions that form our cultural identities. A cultural system based on a worldview built on both the value of the self and the value of our greater essence is foundational in finding balance in our lives and therefore society. It is also, in a sense, the foundation of a healthy democracy.

We must center the systems of the self to optimize our mental and physical health and build the systems within our society that will maximize awareness of our greater essence within it—that is, manifest greater peace and harmony throughout our civilization through connection and balance. But this transformation is likely to be met with great interference, both from within and without—ourselves and our environment.

We are genetically predisposed to react to the reality imposed on us by our environment. From the moment we are born, our worldviews are being shaped by the internal and external environments we experience—birth, hunger, family, friends, education, television, danger, joy, stress, fear, and so on. Through the shaping of our worldviews and cultural identities, our environment helps to construct our reality. The food we eat, the social gatherings we attend, and the economic class that we are told defines us, serve to focus and direct the very energy that we are into the lives that we live—because energy follows consciousness, and consciousness creates reality. Experiences and the symbols that represent them shape our thoughts, and we are what we think. Memories and emotions energize thoughts and activate behavior.

Much of this is the ebb and flow of nature, but much is by human design. The Few and those who cooperate with them know that in its most naked state, power is control of energy, not just the energy that powers our cars, homes, and militaries but also, more importantly, the energy that we, the human race, collectively represent. Control of reality achieves the control of energy, because energy follows consciousness. Those who control the information that we have access to control our reality and therefore, control us. Control of information is a second pillar of power. Can we defend ourselves from this imposed reality?

A tremendous number of resources are being steered into creating our reality. Research has shown that the brain becomes highly receptive to suggestion while watching television (Krugman 1971). Perhaps this is true with all the screens (e.g., computers, smart phones) we are now interfacing with? Commercials and mainstream news programs suggest that it is good to plant GMO seeds for our foods and dump pesticides on our soil. Commercials not only tell us what to buy, but present symbols that enforce beliefs and assumptions about the world and our place in it. Television programming tells us what styles to emulate, clothes to wear, cars to drive. We are taught that happiness is consumerism. Our media tell us what groups to blame for our misery and fear and even sometimes outright pressure us to retaliate against them through our votes and policy approval. Of course, rarely will you see the Few included in these groups to be blamed. The music we listen to, the movies we watch, and the books we read all direct our consciousness. More and more, these messages appear to have ulterior motives driven by the Few, and all of these motives emerge from worldviews built solely on the value of the self.

More alarming is the emerging psychological environment that all this represents and that we find ourselves in. The reality of modern society, with all its beauty and advanced technologies, carries with it poison in the forms of stress, alienation from friends and family (diminishing community), and foods that are both addicting and facilitators of disease and mental and emotional deficit. More and more, society encroaches on our anonymity through infringements on Fifth Amendment rights: corporate and government-sponsored NSA data searches and the Patriot Act. We are very slowly being crushed by fear of coercion by employers, and by major corporations that seem to have an omnipotent presence in government, and by government laws that incrementally erode our liberty, such as allowing our property to be seized (eminent domain) and permitting citizens to be arrested and detained indefinitely without charges, even killed, without due process. These tactics, along with tight control of information via vast media conglomerates, are similar to those used in controlling the minds of cult members. How can we remain balanced under such circumstances?

The value of the self is what drives economies. On the value of the self, great civilizations rise and fall. The value of the self is one wing of human society, but without the value of our greater essence serving as the other wing, society is ultimately unable to soar to the heights of human potential. When society is imbalanced, it is prone to war. A worldview built solely on the value of the self presents great spiritual imbalance. It produces great structural imbalance in society. It breeds imbalanced thinking—a worldview limited to selfishness.

Selfishness leads to imbalance of resources, imbalanced treatment of the environment, imbalanced treatment of the weak and of the "other"—and it leads to war. But perhaps most importantly, the value of the self, left unchecked, has led to the rise of mega-entities that control and disseminate imbalanced information on a transglobal scale. This imbalanced information corrals us into worldviews that focus our energy toward facilitating unimaginable material empires for those who have mastered the implementation of selfishness and who are driven by unquenchable desires to have and consume all things living and dead. As with all greatly imbalanced systems in nature, destruction is sure to follow. To the extent that we are a part of that system, we will fall with it.

If we are to find our balance, we must escape the psychological controls designed to steer our energy toward constructing a reality where unbalanced power can only be the result—where conflict, misery, and disease reign. Escaping these psychological controls involves balancing ourselves holistically.

The first step in regaining our center is fundamental: we strive continuously to realize our greater essence—our connection to all things. We put our lives and all life in perspective. Energy is eternal and cannot be destroyed. We are all immortal in the deepest sense. All things are energy, and although from our perspective we may face chaos and destruction, there is a greater reality—a truer reality of complete harmony and perfect peace underneath it all. We experience this reality when we deeply realize it exists.

Realizing our greater essence is, in a sense, to experience a form of enlightenment. That is, we experience a great insight into the nature of being. The more we practice realizing our greater essence, the more in touch with our creative and intuitive self we become. We become in touch with great peace and the deep joy that arises from the harmony deep within all things. This harmony heals us emotionally and consequently helps to heal us physically. When a critical mass of human beings achieves this state of consciousness, society will become transformed.

We can realize our greater essence while meditating, or praying, or on a hike through the wilderness. We can realize our greater essence while observing the innocence of a child or in our car on the way to work. We can realize our greater essence when someone speaks unkindly about us, or when we engage those who have hurt us in the past. The more we practice, the greater range of circumstances in which we are able to realize the existence of our greater essence, until our consciousness is routinely centered on it in all we do. But there will be interference. We will experience an ebb and flow of connecting with peace as we are caught in the disturbance of falling off our center. If our nature tends to be depressed, for example, we will likely always ebb toward this focus, but can gain greater and greater control throughout our lives. Such change could affect not only our biology but also the actual structure of our brain and even the expression of our DNA (see Richards and Martin 2012).

Anything that impedes our ability to construct a reality centered on the value of our greater essence in balance with the value of the self is interference. The value of the self is epitomized in the selfish gene (selfish memes included). The value of the greater essence is characterized by our connection to all things—harmony, oneness, peace, and love. Interference is the loss of balance within a system of the self (e.g., cognitive, nervous system, digestive system, skeletal system) or our environment. When our center is disturbed, the constructive flow of energy is impeded.

Energy takes on many forms, both measurable and nonmeasurable. This includes the energy created by the body through metabolism and hormonal release, as well as through *chi*. Chi is currently identified as a nonmeasurable energy force, according to martial arts and ancient healing systems from the East such as acupuncture. Balancing the systems of the self is about clearing interference of the energies that empower our lives here on Earth. This interference takes many forms: psychological diversions, negative emotional experiences, damaging worldviews, drug abuse, unhealthy dietary habits, lack of physical conditioning, and even our genetics. Interference can impede our relationship with our environment (family, work), leading to conflict, as well as deficient in the systems of our bodies, leading to pain, disease, and our early demise. Interference can impede our cognitive processes, negatively affecting our abilities to make sound decisions. It can as well affect our emotional health and impede our spiritual direction.

All the systems of a human being are connected and affect one another. If we clear interference from our emotional self, it helps heal our bodies. It is also true that if we clear interference in a system of our body such as the nervous system, it will help us clear interference in our minds. However, this works in reverse as well; that is, if we have interference in one system of the self, a rippling from the disturbance can eventually negatively affect all other systems.

Having a worldview is necessary for us to function throughout our lives, and we are not meant to all have the same worldview. Conflicting worldviews are a part of being human: it is how we respond to the diversity among us that matters most. Entrenched worldviews based solely on the value of the self interfere with realizing our greater essence in all we do.

Worldviews typically emerge as a part of a group identity. Groups and group identity, according to Jonathan Haidt (2012), tend to bind individuals together and also blind those individuals to not only the perspectives of others but sometimes the very humanity of those outside the group. Included in our systems of beliefs and assumptions about the world are the individuals and groups that threaten our worldview. We develop subconscious responses to them, and whenever we become aware of their presence (physically or memetically), we behave accordingly. The response is automatic. It is like a button is pushed in our psyche, and we react with varying levels of defense and hostility that tend to short-circuit our ability to make connections with those who threaten our worldviews and thus impede our ability to solve common problems. These buttons can be used to control us politically because they can quickly disengage our rational minds, leaving us like sheep to be herded by our anger or fear. The subconscious responses we develop toward those who threaten our worldviews also serve to shut off our ability to relate to them, making it easier to convince us that they are worthy of dehumanization. Words that symbolize the "bogymen" that threaten our worldviews are like dog-whistles that call us to action or nonaction with implicit authority. They are used, in a sense, to enslave us, and therefore dehumanize us as well. They make us robot-like in our response to others and their ideas.

To the extent that others can instill in us anger and fear, or associate pain with the bogymen that threaten our worldviews, they help to entrench and empower our subconscious reactions to those they would pit against us. When we are sufficiently threatened, we avoid diverse perspectives altogether and seek out self-validation (i.e., our worldviews) in the television news programs (right or left leaning) we watch, the people we talk to, and the things we read. Fear and anger dash the motivation to examine a wide range of opposing views and facts that could be instrumental in solving the problems that confront us. These activities that we are compelled to engage in, at the expense of understanding multiple perspectives, serve to further divide us and divert us from solving the problems facing our society. It is a powerful psychological prison—one that we cannot always avoid if we want to participate in society. What can we do to escape this trap while remaining fully engaged in our society?

One of the things we can do to liberate ourselves from a robot-like existence is to learn to respond instead of react to our internal and external environments. This skill can serve to deprogram us: freeing us from being activated by those who control information in our society, as well as individuals who know how to press our buttons.

The difference between responding and reacting is cerebral versus emotional. Responding requires analysis and reflection, sometimes even research and planning. Reacting blocks out rational thinking and is knee-jerk in nature: it is characterized by anger, sadness, hopelessness, fear, envy, and pride, as well as blind enthusiasm. Reacting is where the presocial mind lives. By reacting, we are at greater risk of channeling our energies into doing things that we will regret and that undermine our self-interest (not to mention our efforts to create a healthy democracy). Responding instead of reacting is not easy to achieve in all cases; in fact, sometimes it is impossible (in some cases, an intuitive reflex reaction is the best we can hope to achieve, given severe time constraints). But overall, it is possible to respond to our internal as well as external environment as opposed to solely reacting to them. With commitment and practice, we become more adept at responding, and consequently we achieve more self-determination. Even reflexes can become self-programmed. In time, we experience authentic liberty.

Responding requires reflection. When we feel the rise of reaction to a circumstance, we pause and reflect on what is really going on at a deeper psychological level, both internally and externally. We witness our thoughts and feelings. We might also ask what the ideal outcome of a given situation would be. How could that ideal outcome be achieved? We ascertain the facts, make a plan to achieve the ideal outcome, and then decide on the best course to implement the plan (this could happen in a matter of moments or months). Through this process, we transform emotional reaction into rational response. We take unfocused energy and focus it constructively. In yoga philosophy, this involves "seeing clearly, intending, and acting."

We can build much of our lives around the process of seeing clearly, intending, and acting. Our environment continuously requires response. Our responses are based on our perceptions of the events we experience. How we see the events of our lives makes all the difference in world in how we respond: what we think, what we say, and what we do. We are what we think, say, and do; therefore, based on our perceptions, we create who we are. Consequently, there is great power in how we perceive the events of our lives. To the extent that we are the locus of our perceptions, we shape not only our lives, but also reality.

Often in our daily activities, we are required to be strategic planners. We plan our businesses, our meetings, and our day of chores. But we fail to commit the same level of planning toward making ourselves better that we give to implementing our work. Many of us will strive to create total quality in the products and services we sell or deliver, but fail to pursue total quality in our lives. William Glasser (1995) was the first to describe the concept of a *quality world*. Each of us has a quality world, which essentially means the things we hope to receive from interacting with our environment.

Centering the systems of the self is about creating and sustaining quality in all aspects of our lives: spirituality, decision-making and problem solving, emotions, health and fitness, and so on. By building quality in all aspects of our lives, we can create a total quality world around us—a reality of quality living. But what is meant by quality?

Quality is the realization of satisfaction. It is happiness with a given experience. Positive psychology would suggest that happiness is ultimately found in our relationships, caring acts, meaningful endeavors that cause flow (i.e., rapid passing of time), contributing one's strengths to society as well as being fit, positive, and spiritually engaged. These are the seven benchmarks on the path to happiness. A total quality world means finding satisfaction in our spiritual life, our contributions to society. It also means finding satisfaction with our health and our relationships and interactions with others. Centering the systems of the self provides the foundation for constructing our total quality worlds—that is, creating a high level of happiness with our experiences in these areas of our lives by constructively addressing interference that may plague the system(s) of the self. Planning can help us to achieve these important goals.

Identifying our goals is the first step to planning. Goals are based on values. Values are both innate and learned. Understanding our self and our various points of view on any issue that impacts our goals is important to achieving them. Interferences are circumstances that serve as barriers to achieving our goals for wellness—which is the foundation for our quality worlds.

We can successfully pursue a quality world through a rational approach. With an open mind, we can examine the strengths and weaknesses of opposing sides for any issue at hand that may affect our pursuit of wellness in our self and environment. This is key, because most of us will tend to seek out the validation for what we already comfortably believe and, consequently, miss out on opportunities to have a clearer understanding of how to navigate our environment in pursuit of our happiness and a better world. This requires understanding ourselves in relation to our environment. Then, if the values that we base our goals on are balanced between the value of our greater essence and the value of the self, our goals will be better positioned to pursue peace/harmony/oneness/love and quality in our health, our relationships, and our contributions to society. In this way, we create balanced plans for the self that achieve satisfaction with the most important experiences of life—and consequently, we experience happiness. We experience a more profound sense of self-affirmation. According to University of Minnesota researcher Kathleen D. Vohs (2009), self-affirmation not only boosts self-control, it also helps to focus us on what matters most in our lives. Clarity leads to self-awareness, which leads to self-affirmation, and in turn to the things that matters most in life.

On a moment-to-moment basis, seeing clearly, intending, and acting is a planning cycle that we can employ. When our plans are geared to address passing interference such as a rude person who angers us or a common workplace mistake that embarrasses us, we can start by viewing these interferences through the lens of our greater essence. This would mean acknowledging that our pain is due to our limited view of the reality, and this is the first step in seeing clearly. We follow up by analyzing the problem and making a determination of the ideal or best *possible* outcome for the self while maintaining our connection to our greater essence. We then determine our approach to clearing the interference or otherwise pursuing our goals. With our intentions clear, we act or respond. For dealing with greater interference or setting long-range goals that require more thought to address, we can extend this concept to planning, doing, checking, and acting (the PDCA cycle). This is a total quality concept inspired by the work of Edwards W. Deming (1990). It was created for improving organizational systems, but is just as applicable to improving the systems of the self.

Essentially, with the PDCA cycle we identify our goals, plan our response (clearing interference, strengthening the seven behaviors for establishing happiness, and so on), check or evaluate how our plans are working, and then adjust or change them as needed. Finally, we act or respond accordingly with the modified approach in mind.

Planning, acting, and then evaluating our actions establishes control of our consciousness. Power is control of energy. To control human energy, we need to control consciousness. Control of consciousness creates reality because energy follows thought. If we defer to the Few and grant to those who cooperate with them the power to define the meaning of our total reality, we grant them total power. If we control our interpretation of our lives, we gain greater control of our lives.

The first step in liberating ourselves (mind, body, soul, and consequently political self) is to establish our own reality. This doesn't mean hiding our heads in the sand; it means broadening our vision of what we see in the world to include greater spiritual interpretation and a deeper understanding of the motivations driving those who wish to manipulate our reality. By doing so, we erect a second pillar of power in our life—the control of information. When we control the information, assimilate it into our worldview we are in a better position to effectively respond to our environment as opposed to reacting in a robot-like manner to external stimuli. To achieve this, we must maintain sight of our greater essence as our selfish nature pursues a quality world.

From controlling the information that is directed toward our consciousness, either through pursuing our own education or re-interpreting the propaganda directed at us, new structures for the control of information can emerge. These structures can be regular dinner with family that includes discussions on everything from work or school, to wellness, politics, recreation, or spirituality. Regular coffee chats with others about bettering the neighborhood or participating in local government is another possible emergent structure. Structures to control information can also include developing social networks to be aware of legitimate alternative news sources, or creating neighborhood councils, or lobbying local media. Independent or group readings of the Constitution, Bill of Rights, and the Declaration of Independence would be pivotal if it occurred widely. These are not long works of writing. When you see policies that are not consistent with these documents, not only challenge your representatives, challenge your social network to challenge their representatives. It's not hard to Google who your representatives are.

A healthy democracy requires a healthy populace from whom leadership will emerge. A healthy populace is contingent, in part, on the people realizing how easy it is for those who control the apparatus of power to control the human mind and manipulate the people into supporting policies and actions that destroy them and those they love most. When the people can manage the propaganda that the institutions and political class deploy to divide them, they will make political decisions that benefit their own daily lives and those of their loved ones, as opposed to focusing on decisions that hurt those that they fear—based on what our divisions dictate. They will also demand representatives who are passionate about improving their daily lives and the lives of the people they love. Our daily lives and the people we love most are what can unite us as a people and provide our communities with the bimodal symmetry necessary to encourage healthy democracy throughout the nation.

CHAPTER 7

Centering the Heart

The mind cannot stay focused if the heart is scattered.

OUR EMOTIONS CAN be a spiritual power capable of changing the world. Our emotions can also drive deeply evil deeds. In either case, emotions are manifestations of deep reservoirs of energy. The focus of these reservoirs of energy is shaped by our interaction with the environment in which we reside as well as our interpretation of the meaning of ourselves in relationship to this environment. The effect of our environment on our bodies can impact our biology in ways that shape our emotions. For example, not only do physical environmental encounters resulting in concussions produce anger and depression—there is evidence that emotional encounters such as abuse can affect the very structures of our brains (see Kendall 2002). Since our nervous system relates to our glandular system, many also believe that trauma to our spinal alignment can affect the nervous system's role in producing hormones that affect our emotions. Moreover, our environment in large part, activates our genetics. Fight or flight, a most basic biological activity, is a genetic response to environmental factors.

Learned negative perceptions and past negative experiences can become deeply ingrained in our subconscious selves and cause emotional imbalance in our lives. If associated with deep emotions such as fear or anger or lust, these experiences and learned perceptions can become reservoirs of negatively charged energy that can erupt as reactions or become the motivation behind destructive behaviors. We see these behaviors play out in the burning of mosques or destruction of Jewish graveyards, mass shootings from the political right, and the riots that erupt from the political left.

If we want to build a more just world, we must create more justice in our own lives, and to do this, we must clear the way to greater connection with others. Many emotions that operationalize our behaviors can stand in the way of this quest. Not just obvious emotions such as greed, hate, and contempt for the other, but also fear, arrogance, and sloth. Any time our emotions convince us to behave in a manner that dehumanizes or allows for the dehumanization of others, we are blinded from seeing our greater essence—our connection to all things—and we lose our sense of connection that affords others justice. Ultimately, we diminish justice for ourselves.

The great spiritual teachings of the world have tried to guide humanity down a path that steers us clear of these reservoirs of negative emotional energy and the behaviors they spawn through offering moral foundations to live by. These spiritual teachings have strived to define the meaning of life, in part, as our ability to connect in solidarity with one another. These foundations for human reality and consequently human behavior include Hinduism, Buddhism, Judaism, Taoism, Christianity, and Islam, among the many spiritual traditions the world over.

In the West, Christianity and Judaism have served as the primary source of ultimate truth (along with science, of course). These two of the three monotheisms are the foundation of Western morality. Islam, the third monotheism is also a part of this foundation, as is Greek philosophy. Over the last several decades, Eastern moral belief systems have become more influential with regard to Western moral foundations. Fundamental to these theologies and philosophies are the concepts of sin, redemption, and virtue. The *Catechism* of the Catholic Church (1995, 505) defines sin as follows:

> Sin is an offence against reason, truth, and right conscience; it is failure in genuine love for God and neighbor caused by a perverse attachment to certain goods. It wounds the nature of man and injures human solidarity. It has been defined as an utterance, a deed, or a desire contrary to the eternal law.

Papum, the Hindu word for sin, describes behavior that develops negative *karma*. Karma, briefly, is the effect of past actions (of current or former lives) that impact our spiritual attainment. Sin in Hinduism, besides creating negative karma, is the violation of moral and ethical codes. This violation of moral codes is also the view held by the religions of Judaism, Christianity, and Islam. Similarly, the Buddhism and Taoism warning against certain behaviors in many ways parallel the monotheistic idea of sin as being a barrier to spiritual attainment. According to the *Catechisms of the Catholic Church* (1995, 507) there are different kinds of sin.

> When the will sets itself upon something that is of its nature incompatible with the charity [i.e., love] that orients man toward his ultimate end, then the sin is mortal by its very object . . . But when the sinner's will is set upon something that its nature involves a disorder, but is not opposed to the love of God and neighbor, such as thoughtless chatter or immoderate laughter and the like, such sins are venial.

Another important category of sin is *capital sin*. The capital sins are pride, greed, envy, anger, lust, gluttony, and sloth. "A sin is also 'capital' if it is the reason for committing other sins" (Schimmel, 1997, 26).

Pride is human arrogance that puts self before God and neighbor. It is a perceived superiority over others. Cultures all over the world warn against the evils of pride. Greek literature depicts the folly of pride in the story of Icarus, who, despite the warnings of his father, flew too high, causing the sun to melt his wings of wax. In Judaic lore, the story of Adam and Eve depicts pride-driven disobedience of God in eating the forbidden fruit (Schimmel 1997).

In Hindu ethics, pride in achievement is a misguided response to natural forces or a *reaction*, as opposed to a response: "actions are performed by the three forces of nature [prakrti], but, deluded by self-attribution, one thinks, "I did it!" But he who knows the principles that govern the distribution of those forces and the actions, knows that the forces are operating on the forces, and he takes no interest in actions" (Perret 1998, 19). Islam concurs: "Islam condemns pride and self-righteousness, since Almighty God is the only judge of human righteousness" (*The Deen Show* n.d.).

Joseph A. Loya, Wan-Liho, and Chang-Shin Jih in their book *The Tao of Jesus* (1998, 22) quoted Lao Tsu:

> The [general] achieves the objective and stops. But dares not seek to dominate the world; Achieves the objective without bragging; Achieves the objective without boasting; Achieves the objective without arrogance.

According to Michael Schimmel (1997, 57):

> Envy is the pain we feel when we perceive another individual possessing some object, quality, or status we do not possess... It is related to our pride and our quest for recognition, or, for some of us, for fame, glory, and power. When the person is unable to get what he desires, he usually hopes that the person he envies will lose the desired thing and he may even conspire to make that happen.

In Hindu ethics, envy is symptomatic of attachment to materialism, and without such attachment, it is believed that we are free of earthly bondage and consequently enjoy spiritual obtainment. Perret provided some examples of the Hindu ethic in this regard:

"Renunciation is thus rendered compatible with activism. The ideal is the sage all of whose undertakings are devoid of an intention to achieve an object of desire, a being in the world but not of it." (Perret 1998, 19). And "Contented with anything that comes his way, beyond the pairs of opposites, without envy, and equable in success and failure he is not bound, even though he acts" (16).

Both pride and envy, according to Schimmel, are derived from a false sense of self, the former of superiority and the latter of inferiority. Anger is also known as rage, ire, resentment, indignation, vengeance, and wrath. According to Schimmel, Aristotle, Seneca, and Pluto would describe anger as follows: "Anger is aroused when a person suffers a real or perceived injury. Usually the angered person directs his actions towards punishing the real or perceived offender." (Schimmel 1997, 87). Schimmel also noted that "anger is summoned by pride and envy as well as greed and lust. Christian, Judaic, and Islamic lore describe many accounts of anger as counter to spiritual attainment." For example, when Moses lost his temper when the Israelites complained of thirst, he was denied entry to the promisedland. Jesus called for his followers to practice the opposite emotion of anger: "When someone strikes you on the cheek, turn the other one to him as well" (Mt. 5:38-39). Lao Tsu said, "'Repay resentment with virtue" (Loya et al. 1998, 88). Buddha also echoed this sentiment: "If anyone should give you a blow with his hand, with a stick, or with a knife, you should abandon any desires and utter no evil words" (*Majjhima Nikaya* 21.6).

In Hindu ethics, anger is always a reaction. This reaction has two results—obviously the angered person's immediate gratification of unleashing the anger (*phala*), and also building a propensity to repeat that anger (*samskara*). This cycle of repeating reactive behavior is the basis of karma. Hindus seek to transcend the cycle of karma in order to achieve a greater spiritual existence (Perret 1998).

Lust is "the unrestrained and unethical expression of the sexual impulse" (Schimmel 1997, 111). "Lust in Islam is best understood as a lack of temperance that leads one astray from Allah" (Booth 2017,

1). Buddhism also prohibits adultery: "Abstain from unchastity" (Borg 1998, 31). In the Judaic tradition, prohibitions affecting lust were designed to control an otherwise obligatory and enjoyable function of marriage. Cicero, Aristotle, and Plato were wary of the power of lust over humankind. Cicero likened it to madness. But all agreed that it could be controlled (Schimmel 1997).

In Hindu ethics, the impact of lust on spiritual perfection is managed by harmonizing impulsive desire that is unethical with desire that is ethical. For example, a man could have an impulsive lust for a woman outside his marriage as a first-order desire. He also has an ethical desire to be chaste in his marriage, which is his second-order desire. To maintain his ethical will, he must not allow lust to override his second-order desire or he loses his freedom to *act*, as he might prefer. The ideal could be to learn to lust after his wife (Perret 1998, 23-24).

Gluttony in the common sense means to overeat and drink. Schimmel (1997, 12) expounded as follows: "St. Thomas defines gluttony as 'an immoderate appetite in eating and drinking. . . .We regard an appetite as immoderate when it departs from the reasonable order of life in which moral good is found." The opposing virtue of gluttony is temperance or abstinence: doing without food under the regulation of reason. Judaism and Islam closely follow St. Thomas' definition. Along with Aristotle, the three monotheisms prescribe moderated consumption in food and drink, beyond which lies gluttony or, at the other end of the extreme, deprivation.

The Taoist philosophy that calls for moderate behavior in all things supports this view of gluttony:

> The world is a sacred vessel; it may not be mishandled. Whoever covets it will lose it. Therefore among things, some walk ahead, some follow behind; some blow hot, some blow cold; some are strong, some are weak; some are at peace, some are endangered. Accordingly, the Sage discards extremes, extravagance, and excess. (Loya et al. 1998)

Greed is an excessive desire for economic gain and materialism. Greed is motivated by other vices such as envy, gluttony, lust, and pride. Sometimes insecurity (or fear) drives greed. Schimmel (1997, 170) described how the three monotheisms strongly renounce greed:

> The biblical prophets Elijah, Isaiah, Jeremiah, Amos, and Micah were passionate critics of greed and the injustices to which it led. They had the courage and conviction to confront kings and priests when they abused their power and stole from the weak.

The great religions of the East also strive against greed. For example, in Hindu ethics, the effect of greed can be an impediment to escaping the bondage of karma. Taoism and Buddhism prescribe the need to transcend greed to achieve a higher spirituality.

> The Sage desires no-desire,
> Prizes not rare goods, learns to unlearn,
> Redeems the errors of the masses,
> In order to assist the natural spontaneity
> Of the Ten Thousand Things without daring to act [in excess].
> (Loya et al. 1998, 154)

> Riches make most people greedy, and so are like caravans lurching down the road to perdition. Any possession that increases the sin of selfishness or does nothing to confirm one's wish to renounce what one has is nothing but a drawback in disguise. (Borg 1997, 170)

The final capital sin is *sloth*. Sloth is popularly defined as physical laziness, but according to Schimmel (1997, 193) it is much more: "The sin of sloth has two components—*acedia*, which means a lack of caring and aimless indifference to one's responsibilities to God and to man, and *tristitia*, which means sadness and sorrow." The opposite of sloth would be passionate service to neighbor and God—exuberant, joyous commitment to virtuous behavior. Acedia leads to a lack of service to God (transcendent reality), without which there cannot be spiritual attainment. It also means lack of social responsibility.

Each spiritual system requires a search for meaning and motivation for living a spiritual life. Apathy and depression are counterintuitive to the spiritual quest for fulfillment and the betterment of this world. Whether it is Hinduism, Taoism, Buddhism, or the monotheisms, zeal is required for successfully navigating through the barriers Christians know as sin. Without zeal, there can be no spiritual achievement.

At the core of the existence of the great spiritual systems of the world lies the recognition that human beings tend to act in ways inconsistent with a greater spiritual law, as well as the idea that there is hope for redemption. Only though redemption can humanity steer itself away from barriers to our greater essence—nirvana, God, love! *Webster's New World Dictionary* (1976) defined redemption as "repurchase; recover; salvation." Salvation, according to the great religions of the world, is found in faith.

> My own observation, as a historian of religion, would echo this statement: "insofar as he or she has been saved, the Muslim has been saved by Islamic faith; the Buddhist by Buddhist faith, the Jew by Jewish . . . just as Christians have been saved by faith of a Christian form" (Cantwell Smith 1963, 168).

Faith is a theological virtue. It is the common denominator of religions. Not only is faith a virtue, the practice of faith requires virtue. According to *Dictionary.com* (2017), faith can be defined as "Complete trust or confidence in someone or something . . . a strongly held belief or theory." Considering this definition, even an atheist can have complete confidence in the profound connections between self and nature (including all humanity). The potential reverberation that our actions have on others, our environment, and consequently ourselves through the law of cause and effect is something that we all can be conscious of. Complete confidence in such a theory beckons us to pursue virtuous behavior even if this form of faith is not theological.

The *Catechism of the Catholic Church* (1995, 495) describes virtue as follows: "Human virtues are firm attitudes, stable dispositions, habitual perfections of intellect and will that govern our actions, order our passions, and guide our conduct according to reason and faith." According to the *Catechism*, categories of virtues include *theological* and *cardinal* virtues. In addition to faith, the other theological virtues are *hope* and *charity*. Through hope we aspire to dwell in heaven, to be with God. Charity is how we love God and our fellow human beings.

The *Catechism* states that the cardinal virtues are *prudence, justice, fortitude*, and *temperance*, and describes these virtues as follows: Prudence is "the virtue that disposes practical reason to discern our true good in every circumstance and to choose the right means of achieving it." Justice "disposes one to respect the rights of each and to establish in human relationships the harmony that promotes equity with regard to persons and to the common good." Fortitude is "the moral virtue that ensures firmness in difficulties and constancy in the pursuit of the good." Finally, temperance is "the moral virtue that moderates the attraction of pleasures and provides balance in the use of created goods."

Striving to avoid spiritual transgressions, to achieve virtuous behavior and maintain faith, are commonalities of the great spiritual systems of the world. Schaefer (1994, 3) described other commonalities of the religions of the world:

> That which we call God is justice, love, compassion and mercy, which are generously poured over humanity; that "man's path to God is one of sacrifice, renunciation, resignation, moral discipline, the via purgativa, prayer and meditation" . . . that man must live on Earth according to certain standards in order to attain salvation in both this life and the life to come; and that the common ethical basis of all religions is

the so-called Golden Rule known to us from the Gospel: "Therefore all things whatsoever ye would that men should do to you, do even so to them." . . . finally, the most fundamental feature common to all religions is mysticism, the highest aim of which is the unity of the soul with the eternal God.

According to Christina Heavrin et al. (1997), ethics is essentially the values and rules humans live by. So what specific values are explicit in the Golden Rule? The Golden Rule is framed by the various religions in slightly different ways:

> Baha'i: "Choose thou for thy neighbor that which thou chosest for thyself." (langleybahai.org, retrieved 2020)
> Islam: "No one of you is a believer until he desires for his brother that which he desires for himself." (Islam.ru, retrieved 2/25/2020)
> Taoism, Lao Tsu: "If one loves the world as one's body, one can be entrusted [to care] for the world." (Loya et al. 1998, 66)
> Hinduism: "This is the sum of true righteousness—treat others as you would yourself be treated." (Templeton 1999, 5)
> Judaism: "What is hateful to you, do not to your fellow man; that is the entire law; all the rest is commentary." (Templeton 1999, 16)
> Buddha: "Consider others as yourself." (Borg 1997, 15)
> Chief Seattle: "We did not weave the web of life, we are merely a strand in it. Whatever we do to the web, we do to ourselves." (Templeton 1999, 92)

The common assumption across these versions of the Golden Rule is that there are ways, or a way, that we as humans want (in common) to be treated. Which, of course, begs the question: how do human beings want other human beings to treat them?

It seems it is common that humans want to be accepted by other human beings (preferably unconditionally). Humans want to be forgiven when they have wronged others. Humans want compassion when they are wounded; they want understanding. Humans want other humans to care about them—their rights, their needs, their lives. Humans want to be treated as if loved.

What we want from others is love—unconditional love.

The Golden Rule is the law, but the goal is agape love. "Agape love is unlimited, pure, and unconditional. It is an altruistic love, given for its own sake without expecting anything in return. Aspiring to agape love is not exclusive to any one religion, but is an underlying principle in all major world religions" (Sir John Templeton 1999).

Unconditional love is a natural phenomenon among humans. We love our children when they are sick and when they are in good health, whether they grow up to be rich or poor, sinful or virtuous. We love our children unconditionally, perhaps because they are who we are—a part of us that shall carry on long after our deaths. We love our parents too, because they are us. Without them we would not exist. We love siblings because they share the genetic history and the upbringing that contributes to who we are. They also, as part of our upbringing, helped to create us. Our siblings are a reflection of who we are because of our common origin. We love our spouses too: for richer or for poorer, in sickness and in health. We love them despite their imperfections. Spouses share their lives; they build one life together and make decisions together; they share their bodies and their emotions. Spouses share their thoughts and values. They share their time here on Earth. Our spouses reflect who we are, as do our friends. Our friends usually have the same values, same interests, same social class, usually the same race and religion. In these commonalities that draw us together, our friends too are us.

> Confucianism would hold that all forms of love are inseparable parts of the same fabric. In other words, there is a relationship between the way mayors and governors carry out

their civic responsibilities and the way they treat their spouses and their sons and daughters. It is all a part of the same web of love (Sir John Templeton 1999, 85).

The ability to see ourselves in others is an essential part of the journey toward residing in a state of agape love. To recognize the commonality of our humanity and the humanity of others despite our many differences is key to opening the door to agape love. But to *feel* the humanity of others is to cross over from isolation into the unity provided only by love. Empathy is the threshold to agape love.

The Unitarian minister S. Alexander said in a sermon (2004) that the English word *empathy* comes from the Greek word *empatheia*, which literally means "feeling into." According to Alexander,

> Empathy, then, at its most fundamental level, is the quality of feeling into the lives and struggles and circumstances of others. It is an emotional merging of your humanness with that of another . . . it is a direct, heartfelt sense of belonging (with others) that allows you to reach out to them in compassion, connection, and concern.

The universal value is agape love: its law is the Golden Rule, and its vehicle is empathy. Virtue, sin, and redemption are all about the quest for agape love and its expression. As we read in I Corinthians 13:

> I may be able to speak the language of men and even of angels, but if I have no love, my speech is no more than a noisy gong or a clanging bell. I may have the gift of inspired preaching; I may have all knowledge and understand all secrets; I may have all the faith needed to move mountains—but if I have no love, I am nothing. I may give away everything I have, and even give up my body to be burned—but if I have no love, this does me no good.

Love is patient and kind; it is not jealous or conceited or proud; love is not ill mannered or selfish or irritable; love does not keep a record of wrongs; love is not happy with evil, but is happy with the truth. Love never gives up; and its faith, hope and patience never fail.

Love is eternal. There are inspired messages, but they are temporary; there are gifts of speaking in strange tongues, but they will cease; there is knowledge, but it will pass. For our gifts of knowledge and of inspired messages are only partial; but when what is perfect comes, then what is partial will disappear.

When I was a child, my speech, feelings, and thinking were all those of a child; now that I am a man, I have no more use for childish ways. What we see now is like a dim image in a mirror; then we shall see face to face. What I know now is only partial; then it will be complete—as complete as God's knowledge of me.

Meanwhile these three remain; faith, hope, and love; and the greatest of these, is love.

CHAPTER 8

Balancing the Heart with the Mind

An Old Cherokee told his grandson, "My son, there is a battle between two wolves inside us all. One is Evil. It is anger, jealousy, greed, resentment, inferiority, lies and ego. The other is Good. It is joy, peace, love, hope, humility, kindness, empathy, and truth." The boy thought about it, and asked, "Grandfather, which wolf wins?" The old man quietly replied, "The one you feed."
--author unknown

IF WE OBSERVE the messages that the Few and those who cooperate with them communicate through corporate and state-sponsored media the world over, we can see how much of it encourages emotional forms of focus that are the barriers to agape love. We are inundated with images and stories shaped to instill perpetual fear (as opposed to hope and faith), perpetual anger and hate, envy, pride, lust, immoderacy, and apathy. All these become reservoirs of negative emotions that erode empathy, our bridge to the one type of unity that is more powerful than the apparatus used by the Few. These barriers are implanted in our minds through commercial advertisements (print, radio, and television) and news sources and entertainment media as well as political parties. Inevitably we participate in the socialization of each other into these frames of thinking. This process that corrupts us is essentially propaganda technique. According to *Wikipedia.com*:

> Propaganda is a specific type of message presentation, aimed at serving an agenda. Even if the message conveys true information, it may be partisan and fail to paint a complete and balanced picture. The primary use of the term is in political context and generally refers to efforts sponsored by governments and political parties [as well as transnational corporations].
>
> The goal of propaganda is either to win support of or defeat a certain position, rather than to simply present the position. The primary target of propaganda is people's opinion, rather than their knowledge. Therefore the information conveyed is often presented in an emotionally loaded way and with other means of affecting the opinions of people.

The position that the Few and their alliances seek to defeat is (in effect) *agape love*.

Edward Barnays (1928, 47, 31, 37), the father of modern propaganda technic wrote:

> If we understand the mechanisms and motives of the group mind, is it not possible to control and regiment the masses according to our will without their knowing?...Small groups of persons can, and do, make the rest of us think what they please...[This] invisable government tends to be concentrated in the hands of the few because of the expense of manipulating the social machinery which controls the opinions and habits of the masses.

Much of the communication by our media and political parties is designed to control our opinions and therefore our minds. Sometimes even so-called scientific research papers contain aspects of propaganda.

Left v Right academics, and so-called "liberal" or "conservative" media outlets and politicians work together, consciously and inadvertently, to steer us into groups at odds with one another. We become the scapegoats sacrificed on the altar of division, while those at odds with our democracy go unscathed. The goal here is to help us recognize this reality so we can become aware of the pervasiveness and potential impact of the propagandized messages that bombard us daily and become empowered to filter out these destructive memes.

The vehicles of propaganda today, such as media of all sorts, political representatives, political parties, and increasingly, educational materials, are powerful delivery systems because they often represent legitimate organizations that play on our frustrations as well as our sense of duty. Legitimate organizations that use propaganda techniques to stir up and direct our frustrations have very powerful effects on how we *feel* about ourselves and others. When the medium of such propaganda is television, we are particularly vulnerable because we are then more susceptible to suggestion. According to the freedictionary.com suggestion can be defined as "the process of inducing a thought, sensation, or action in a receptive person without using persuasion and without giving rise to reflection in the recipient."

The propaganda that promotes our baser instincts like greed, pride, or fear represents an argument for division among the population that in effect conquers empathy and therefore the unity of community shaped by the pursuit of agape love through reciprocal altruistic (win-win) strategies (i.e., our unite and liberate strategy).

Ultimately, the culture of divide and conquer emanates in large part from these media outlets that perpetuate and support political rhetoric and thus policy that follows this same projection. Moreover, the corporate oligarchy relies on being able to activate these reservoirs of negative emotions to induce us to *react* in ways that perpetuate a culture that divides us and accepts and even encourages injustice. We are thereby imprisoned in the darkness that is our separation from realizing our greater essence (oneness/harmony/peace), which is love. Agape is the aligning of the heart with our greater essence, and for many of us, our greater essence is God.

The struggle between perpetuating transgressions against agape and the greater realization of agape in society is an ancient and ongoing one. This struggle calls us, now more than ever, to weigh in. Balancing the heart with the mind is about responding with empathy and understanding instead of reacting to propaganda stimuli based on reservoirs of negative emotions. It is about observing, understanding, and deactivating our own demons instead of letting them be buttons for others to push to control our behavior. We use reflection and understanding to de-energize the presence of our demons and then refocus this energy in more constructive ways. When we achieve this, we free our hearts from the slavery imposed on us by others. We clear away the barriers to empathizing across our divisions, and we realize our greater essence—our connections to all things. Thereby we enter the domain of a power greater than wealth and political apparatus. If God is love, the great spiritual teachings of the world make clear the emotions and behaviors that emanate from us that stand between heaven and hell, not only in the next world, but also here on Earth.

At their roots, Islam, Judaism, Christianity, Buddhism, Hinduism, Taoism, and other spiritual systems discourage the superficial desires for objects and status and instead encourage a focus on striving for altruism based on agape. If we look at our reservoirs of negative emotional energy and prescribed remedies through the lens of the world's great spiritual teachings, we see an incredible consistency. In the great spiritual systems of the world, we find common descriptions of destructive behaviors that stand in the way of our realizing our greater essence (connection to all things: love!) as well as behaviors that promise to liberate all of humankind—prudence, justice, fortitude, faith, and hope. But what do these virtues mean in a practical sense for today's reality?

Without having a belief in a transcendent reality, fear and selfishness promise to be our masters. For some, this transcendent reality is our connection to all things—one ecosystem, one humanity, all energy ultimately connected in complete harmony. For others, it is nirvana; still others call it God. Yet each of these descriptions centers on one great achievement—love—and so the centering of the heart is guided by empathy because empathy leads to connection, and connection leads to love. We therefore become the natural steward of all earthly energy through empathy. We become the stewards of our ecosystems–of humanity, of our own bodies, minds, and souls.

We are human, yes. In the right context and measure, our negative reservoirs of energy can even be constructive. The critical factor is balance. Is our lust, greed, or envy negatively affecting our realization of being connected to all things? Is it negatively affecting our relationships or our health? We cannot be completely free of emotional imbalance while remaining human, but there is hope that we can become better and that our personal evolution will contribute to a greater cultural evolution of humankind. We do this through a process that again builds on seeing clearly, intending, and acting.

I have struggled over the course of my life with a tendency to react to my environment instead of responding. I have been able to make life-transforming gains through learning to see clearly, intending, and acting. In the following I will introduce my framework for achieving these gains. This framework consists of Reflection, Reinterpretation and Reframing, Restoring (realizing my greater essence), Refiling (self-determining my triggers), and finally, Responding (prudence).

I'd like to share with you an incident from my childhood. I didn't realize it at the time, but a little speech from my gym teacher laid out an important foundation for addressing my ability to connect with others despite negative emotions I had toward them.

When I was about nine years old, I was transferred to a new school. The teacher in charge of gym was a former professional soccer player. Most of the kids in the area where I lived knew nothing about soccer, including me. But thanks to this gym teacher, the kids at my new school had been playing the sport for some time. I was among the more athletic kids in my class, but I didn't stand a chance against these guys. They blew past my efforts, leaving me in the dust. This of course enraged me. I often threw tantrums and even started fights. I resented these kids and their "stupid game."

My anger and violent outbursts kept me from connecting with my classmates. After a few games, the gym teacher pulled me aside. He said, "Look, kid, stop and think. You're so mad at everybody, but why? Think how long these kids have been playing soccer compared to you. You think you're doing terrible, but in light of the situation, you're doing pretty good—think of that! You're showing everybody that you're better than most of them were when they first learned the game. The question is are you going to focus on learning the skills of the game or focus on the fact that these guys have better skills than you?"

I did what he asked of me: I reflected, reframed my assessment of myself, and my environment, saw my situation in a new light, and focused on learning the game. I got along much better with the kids after that, and I became a better soccer player, a lot better. I eventually became one of the better players in that school.

Reflection: The Awareness of Self and Environment

Becoming aware of our stored reservoirs of negative emotionalized experiences and perceptions (prejudices, fears, misplaced lust, anger, sloth, and so on) is a lifelong pursuit. Sometimes we need to take the pursuit under professional guidance, such as cognitive behavior therapy. However, most of the time we can, on our own, pursue awareness of these past experiences and learned views by reflecting on our reactions to our environment that are emotional and nonconstructive. Honesty and nonjudgment is essential to the process of self-reflection. This self-reflection process is straightforward. Perhaps we are angry toward others. Could this be in part a biological issue (lack of sleep, stress)? What is the impact of this behavior? How is this anger affecting my health and relationships? You simply need to ask yourself if you are reacting to your environment in an emotionally destructive manner. Is it a matter of a bruised ego (pride) on your part? Is this anger driven by greed or envy? Is this an ongoing pattern of behavior within my life? Am I blaming others inappropriately? Am

I overgeneralizing the behavior of others? Am I obsessing with my point of view? Am I projecting reasons for their behavior that just aren't there? Am I really getting angry with a particular person or a group that has hurt me in the past and that they are associated with? For most of us, through reflection such as this we can begin to see clearly if we are honest with ourselves.

Once we come to honest answers about our reactions and the motivations behind them, we are ready to reinterpret our environment in relationship to ourselves in ways that can change how we feel about others and our place in the world. This change is to be designed to help us see beyond our reservoirs of negative emotion. This new view of our environment and self serves as the basis for new behavior focused on our life goals and desire to better society (at least in our own small realm of influence).

Reinterpretation and Reframing: The Meaning of Self and Environment

It is human nature to make judgments about others based on superficial information. Sometimes such judgment is necessary, but it can also be the motivation behind physically, emotionally, and spiritually diminishing behaviors. It can also inspire misdirected vengeance and horrific violence. Real or perceived injury to ourself or to extensions of ourself, including our worldview, can cause reactions that turn into destructive beliefs and assumptions that can be used as buttons for others to manipulate us. However, once we realize through reflection the existence of such reservoirs of negative emotions, we can, in many cases, begin to transform them with reason.

Let's take, for example, the meme of the *superpredator* perpetually driven home by television news anchors, movies and television shows, pictures in the daily newspapers, and the water-cooler discussions among our co-workers. The meme is clear—this is a criminal who wreaks havoc on society through poisoning our children with drugs, murders indiscriminately, would rape our beloved ones heartlessly, and whose existence is a drain on society. This criminal is young, athletic, dresses in urban styles, *and is a black male (or Hispanic)*. The message of harm is perpetually associated with the superficial description, and through association inevitably becomes one and the same in our minds. That is, young, athletic, and urban-styled black males become synonymous with fear, danger, and perceived injury to our safety, well-being, and worldview. One look at a youth who fits the superpredator meme and we react with fear, anger, and even misdirected vengeance and violence. But is this *really* all that there is to such black males? Certainly, the answer to that question is *no*! But what about the truly hardened gang-bangers, the ones who are convicted and guilty of terrible crimes, aren't they a part of our greater essences?

All of us are the sum of our conscious mind's focus and projections and of our heart's level of freedom to love. We are also subject to our environment's impact on our biology and resultant behavior. Considering these factors, we might also ask how this same constant message about young black males affects the conscious and subconscious minds of young black males. What is the real and perceived injury of this meme on the hearts of these youth and the impact of this stress on their biology? If our bodies are assaulted by the violence and stress associated with poverty, by the poisons of cheap processed foods that dominate local markets in economically depressed areas where so many live (see *Fast Food Genocide*, Fuhrman 2017); if our hearts are assaulted by society's rejection, fear, disdain, and police harassment and brutality—where is this likely to direct the focus of our conscious minds, not to mention our hearts? If we, and those like us, are subjected to dehumanization, aren't we being taught to dehumanize others? The *root causes* of the gang-banger, rather than the gang-banger himself, are the truer or greater threat to our safety, well-being, and worldview. The superpredator meme may not have even been created if the focus had been on the underlying causes of crime as opposed to superficial externalities of certain youth. With these thoughts in mind, we might learn to see the young, athletic, urban-styled black male differently from what the superpredator meme suggests.

Of course, I'm not asking that dangerous criminals, whether they be black, white, rich, or poor, be allowed to victimize anyone. I am, however, suggesting that we learn to better transcend our own psychological victimization in order to see clearly, intend appropriately, and act responsibly. This also means that the same process of reframing could be used by young black males to help themselves transcend the assault on their humanity imposed on them by the superpredator meme. Through reframing, we have the potential to shake off false images of ourselves as well as others and create our own view of being and being-with.

Reinterpreting or reframing can help us escape the many psychological prisons imposed on us by the Few and their alliances. Another example of this can be found in the reframing of the powerful *conspicuous consumption* meme. Our natural desire to be loved can be unconsciously confused with a desire for status. If we can obtain a high status in society (we think subconsciously), we will be admired, and this admiration is confused with being loved. Consequently, we can have the tendency to pursue the trappings of material status because we are inundated with the idea of a person's wealth being synonymous with their status in society (how much others value them). Through conspicuously consuming, we broadcast our status in society, but it is really an unconscious cry for love, and we find only disappointment because we do not find love at all. Consequently, we seek more status and consume more conspicuously. The cycle never ends until we see conspicuous consumption clearly and reframe the meaning of conspicuous consumption to what it is in actuality—a failed attempt at achieving love. Once we do this, it loses its power. We become free of the prison cycle of *more-bigger-better-more* that is used by the Few and their alliances to control our lifelong expenditure of energy. This cycle focuses our consciousness on negative emotions such as envy, pride, and greed. This cycle divides us and destroys the unity necessary to stand against the Few. It isolates us from the very thing we seek—love.

Restoring: Connecting with Our Greater Essence—Love

The goal of Reinterpreting and Reframing is to remove the obstacles to our balanced view of our self and others. When we see beyond the barriers to agape love, we restore our connection to our greater essence. Reframing is successful when it positively affects our self-perceptions, enhances feelings of empathy, improves our relationships, and contributes to our health. To the extent that this is achieved, we are *Restored*. For example, let's say our best friend just bought a new house and it is everything *we* ever wanted and yet don't have. As a result, deep in our hearts, we hope that our friend would experience some problem with their new home purchase. We are envious. "Why isn't that house ours instead?" we might think. We become restored if we can learn to accept our friend's material achievement as something having to do with their own life or fate, see it as "God's will, not mine," and instead focus on our own life. If we can learn to understand that our feeling of inferiority about not having that splendid home is really an illusion, because in the greater reality we are not inferior and our happiness is found internally, then we are better able to restore our pathway to agape love. We become restored through agape love because the realization of agape in our lives creates in us a better biology, more supportive of our own health and more supportive of our relationships. These developments reflect our connection to our greater essence. We balance the heart with the mind, and this takes practice, a lifetime of practice. We may not be able to be perfect in this life, but we can become better—the goal is continuous improvement.

Refiling: Creating New Realities Through Amending Our Worldviews

Eventually, the situation that has caused us to feel envious (for example) looks different to us. It no longer makes us feel inferior because we have stopped allowing it to be a subconscious trigger associated with feelings of inferiority. We simply learn to see it differently. We may also decide to *create a trigger* for positive emotions such as hope or caring. Perhaps our problem is sloth (a lack of caring), and let's say it's about the effects of environmental pollution on certain economically depressed areas. We are not economically depressed and don't see the direct impact of pollution in poor communities on our lives, and so the issue is not immediate for us. Consequently, we lack connection and empathy. Intellectually, we do realize the value of solidarity with these impoverished people, but desire greater motivation to act.

Provided that our life has brought us to the point that we now wish to care more, we can use the processes of Reflection, Reinterpreting and Refiling by interfacing with print, multimedia, lectures, friends, family, or associates who are deeply concerned with how pollution in economically depressed communities affects *our world*. The goal is to make oneself aware of the threat of pollution to the *self* and to those individuals and things that we associate with the self. The more the information threatens us or those we love the greater are the reservoirs of emotional energy created. Once the self develops strong emotions about the effects of human activity on the environment, the more we are apt to be energized, to care—and consequently, connect with others facing a similar threat. Our connection can serve as motivation to address the issue. Ideally, we could also pursue this process by focusing on developing direct connections with the impoverished living in highly polluted environments and thereby enhancing our concerns about the well-being of this particular group in general. What we are trying to do here is build experiences that develop pools of emotional energy that help to motivate us.

As long as the focus of the information we are using to discourage apathy and encourage zeal is also associated with constructive responses, we will likely be more hopeful and responsible in our actions. The point is that we can be the masters of our animation. We simply must commit.

Responding with Love Instead of Reacting with Negativity

Responding with love begins with a question to the self: "How can I make the best of the situation of feeling anger or greed or apathy, or . . .?" If we can reframe our view of our self or those whom we perceive as the cause of our negative emotions in a more humanizing light, we can begin the transformation.

When we analytically reflect on our emotions, we bring them into our rational mind, where they can be reshaped. We then seek to discover not only the origins (past experiences and roots) of these emotions, but more importantly, we discover rational alternative, constructive, humanizing responses to our feelings about ourself and others. Then we practice those responses. By doing this, we begin to reprogram our subconscious responses to emotions and our environment in ways that are more responsive (as opposed to being reactive).

If we refocus our consciousness, energy will follow, producing new emotions and behavior. Consequently, we are not only shaping ourselves to act more responsibly and effectively, we become more difficult to manipulate. We also open ourselves up to the possibility of self-love, empathy, and agape. As each reservoir of emotion and motivation becomes reframed and redirected, there is one less push-button in animating our behavior for the Few and those who cooperate with them. In essence, we are ridding our lives of the chains that keep us from developing the kind of community that will effectively end their reign. We become more able to fill our lives with gratitude, love, spirituality, and meaning.

This new life focus brings us into the present. It helps establish flow in our work and daily lives as well as our ability to contribute to society in meaningful ways. We are no longer held hostage by past experiences that lock our consciousness on past painful experiences nor on thoughts of a future that shackle us with fear.

We can fill our hearts with fortitude by reassociating triggers that once inspired negative reactions with positive responses instead. We can animate our actions with justice through empathy, and by seeing clearly, we focus our responses with prudence. We can find faith, hope, and love by freeing our hearts of the chains of propagandized suggestions sowed throughout the empires of corporatocracy and totalitarians. When we balance our hearts with our minds, we strengthen our bodies and are better able to build our community with love.

CHAPTER 9

Centering the Systems of the Body

Peace eludes the heart when the body is in turmoil.

Balancing the Body with Our Greater Essence

When I was a small child struggling with violence and health issues, my mother intuited a need for me to begin a journey quite foreign to the Western view of the world at the time. It was a journey into a variety of traditions and techniques that revolved around optimizing the flow of subtle energy through the body and mind. My mother knew that, like most kids, I loved superheroes. One morning she asked me if I would I like to try to develop superhero powers. She said, "Did you know the yogis can emit energy from their hands? It's a healing energy, not a destructive one. But they must practice for a very, very long time to do that. They must first become very, very healthy. Do you want to practice?" I was a little boy who saw his chance to be like a superhero, and I pursued it with all my heart. In time, what I learned was that yoga postures, meditation, *do-in*, *qigong*, certain sounds (chanting), breathing exercises, strength and cardiovascular training, even eating healthy are about creating circumstances in our bodies that allow subtle energy, or *chi*, to freely flow through us and invigorate our lives. This flow of subtle energy that permeates our

Centering the Systems of the Body

bodies and minds bring balance to the systems of the self and helps to optimize our lives here on Earth. It helps us to project balance into the world. According to Cyndi Dale (2009, xx-xxi),

> Underlying physical reality are subtle, or indiscernible energies that create and sustain all matter. The so-called real world—the one you can touch, smell, taste, hear, and see—is constructed entirely from these energies, which are imperceptible through the five senses. In fact, *all of reality is created from organized and changeable systems of subtle energy*. To most effectively help someone heal—aid the sick, alleviate suffering, and bring hope where there is darkness—we must acknowledge and work with the subtle energies that create imbalances and disease . . . The human body is a complex energetic system, composed of hundreds of energetic subsystems. Disease is caused by energetic imbalance; therefore health can be restored or established by balancing one's energies.

Theoretically, there are hundreds of energy structures (depending on the wellness or philosophical–spiritual practice referenced). However, most revolve around three primary energy structures—fields, channels, and bodies. These structures permeate and create our bodies and connect us to the outer world.

All living things, as well as the Earth and the sky, have fields, also known as auras. These fields emanate from us and also draw subtle energy or chi into us. If they are weak, they allow destructive energies such as negative thoughts and emotions to affect us. Our auras connect us to the energy of the Earth and universe (as well as all living things and our greater essence). They help enable our thoughts and attitudes to affect others without our saying or doing anything. Auras are also connected to energy structures within us known as *energy bodies* or *chakras*. The chakras relate to our organs and, through energy streams known as *nadis*, permeate our entire bodies (connective tissue and cells). Larger energy streams (usually known as meridians) with pooling locations (acupuncture–acupressure points) also relate to bodily systems and also help increase the flow of energy throughout our physical self. There appear to be at least four sources of subtle energy:

1) plant and animal life, and water (processed through digestion and distributed through our cardiovascular system),
2) air (processed through our lungs and distributed through our cardiovascular system),
3) sunshine (processed through our skin and distributed through our endocrine system),
4) electromagnetic energy (processed through our auras, chakras, and acupoints and distributed through our nadis and meridians).

When these fields, channels, and bodies of energy are clear of obstructions (negative attitudes, bad experiences, chemical imbalances, structural misalignment, energy blockages), life-building energy permeates our minds and bodies and we experience an elevated level of balance between the self and our greater essence. Consequently, we experience and project more peace, harmony, and love into what we manifest here on Earth. We become physically healthier, and our thoughts become more constructive, as do our words and our deeds. We also become open to greater creativity and intuition because we have a greater connection to all things knowable and unknowable. There are many exercises and practices that are said to clear our bodies and minds of elements that obstruct this flow, some of which I have already offered.

This idea of subtle energies is far from being fully embraced by the Western health and scientific establishment. Nonetheless, researchers such as Dr. James Oschman, Fritz-Albert Popp, and Changlin Zhang (the Zhang-Popp theory (see Dale 2009) and Dr. Bjorn Nordenstrom (see Dale 2009) have conducted research-based theories of energetic systems that offer greater explanation of subtle energy theory. Techniques such as acupuncture, meditation, qigong, and yoga have begun to open the minds of empiricists as to their value on a practical basis. But to date, how they actually work often remains a mystery to science.

My experience with these practices is that of a lay practitioner. I'm not a master instructor or teacher in any of them. I have combined practices offered by those who are masters and qualified instructors to consciously optimize the functions of the fields, channels, and bodies that transfer subtle energies throughout my being. I have practiced for many years. These practices have transformed me from a very negative minded individual headed for destruction to a happy, healthy, and productive human being. I encourage you to seek out qualified instructors for these techniques and do so in consultation with your nutritionist and family practitioner.

Meditation

There are many reputable studies on the positive effects of meditation. Among the best known are anxiety and stress reduction, even relief from depression. But there are many more: calming and balancing the human nervous system reportedly encourages whole brain synchronization, enhances endocrine system function, improves pH balance in the body, and is an aid in strengthening the human bioenergy field (the aura). The healing that can take place with meditation is not just psychological, it is physical and, some contend, even spiritual. Meditation increases GABA and DHEA in the brain, and this is believed to reduce the likelihood of contracting ailments such as cancer and heart disease. With a stronger endocrine system, we are happier and age more slowly. It is believed that with stronger bioenergy fields, we are less affected by the negative attitudes of those around us and we are more in tune with the positive energies of nature and humankind. By helping to synchronize the left and right hemispheres of the brain, meditation helps us to integrate intuition and creativity with analytical–logical thinking to solve the problems we face.

Meditation increases alpha, gamma, theta, and delta wave patterns in the brain. Alpha waves calm the autonomic nervous system and heighten the parasympathetic nervous system (the healing system). Gamma waves reduce fear and support sustained happiness. Theta waves increase creativity and the ability to remember and help with problem solving (traditionalists such as yoga masters believe the third eye is opened with these waves). Finally, delta waves help us to gain access to our unconscious mind (some traditionalists believe they heighten awareness of the paranormal world). Delta waves also occur during deep sleep.

Stress is believed to be the cause of many illnesses. Therefore, we could say that many illnesses start in our minds—our consciousness. Since energy follows consciousness, when our consciousness is entangled in the pain of the past or fear of the future, our consciousness is focused on destructive energies that reverberate throughout our body and stress our nervous and endocrine systems, which can affect our pH balance and immune system. Stress is also said to weaken our bioenergy field (aura). Meditation helps to focus our consciousness on the present as opposed to having it trapped in the past or future. This focus helps to align our consciousness with our state of being deep within ourselves, beyond the chaos of society. We connect with our greater essence and gain a sense of healing through the peace that we find.

From a scientific perspective, there are two types of meditation—*focused* and *open monitoring*. Focused meditation includes the most widely known form of meditation, *mantra meditation*, using sounds like *om* or *aum*, a repetitive chant to help focus consciousness away from thoughts of the past or future. We could use any of numerous other sounds, even the Hail Mary prayer. Most scientists maintain that the specific sound is inconsequential; what matters is the use of an anchor for focusing our attention. The traditionalists (yogic and Hindu practitioners, many aboriginal shamans) disagree and place great significance on particular mantras or chants. For the traditionalists, sound plays a pivotal role in existence. It affects our subtle energy system and consequently our body, mind, and soul.

Some researchers tend to support the views of the traditionalists. The work of Hans Jenny (1967, 1974) suggests that certain sound patterns that interact with vibration can create patterns in reality. He used certain frequencies to create patterns in sand that he could reproduce. Dr. Masaru Emoto, in his book *The Hidden Messages in Water,* describes how he uses sound to shape water crystals (although some question his methodology).

Pjotr Garajajev and Vladimir Poponin have done research presented in their article "DNA BioComputer Reprogramming" that takes the notion of the effect of sound on matter even further. Rex Research Group (2016) described the work of these Russian scientists:

> The most astonishing experiment that was performed by Garajajev's group is the reprogramming of the DNA codon sequences using modulated laser light. From their discovered grammatical syntax of the DNA language they were able to modulate coherent laser light and even radio waves and add semantics (meaning) to the carrier wave. In this way they were able to reprogram in vivo DNA in living organisms, by using the correct resonant frequencies of DNA. . . Our own DNA can simply be reprogrammed by human speech, supposing that the words are modulated on the correct carrier frequencies.

Mantra meditation is just one of the many forms of focus meditation. Some others include *aura meditation, chakra meditation,* and *compassion meditation.* Aura meditation has to do with visualizing the aura as white light and imagining the energy cleansing the body with electromagnetic energy and healing emotions and physical areas of pain. Chakra meditation focuses on a particular chakra (locations along the center of the body) for healing in the parts of the body governed by the chakra; it may use mantras associated with each chakra (*vam* for the first chakra, *lam* for the second, *ram* for the third, *yam* for the fourth, *ham* for the fifth, and *om* for the sixth and seventh chakras), generally balancing the energy of the chakra system. This is said to also cleanse the aura.

Compassion meditation focuses on well-intentions toward self, loved ones, those whom we see neutrally, and finally those we see with negative emotions. The ideal is to reach a state of positive intention toward all equally. Compassion meditation increases self-acceptance as well as empathy for others.

Christian meditation is a process used to obtain moral purification and a profound closeness to Christ–God. It is achieved through contemplating the wisdom of the Bible, repetitive praying such as the Hail Mary, or deeply focusing one's consciousness on being in the presence of God.

Open monitoring meditation is a form of observing without judgment or attachment. Open monitoring meditation includes *mindfulness meditation*. Mindfulness is the process of simply being aware of our internal and external worlds—what we see, hear, feel, smell, and touch. We can be mindful of eating, speaking, and walking. Another form of open monitoring meditation includes *daily life meditation*, which involves reflecting without judgment or attachment on our daily activities. Like all open monitoring meditation, daily life meditation draws us into our present state of being and allows us to better tune into our greater essence.

Meditation is simple to learn, but takes practice to become efficient at it. Books, videos, and instructors abound. Many online sources for learning meditation are free. Its benefits, however, can be truly a treasure.

Breathing Exercises

Focused breathing can be used in meditation. There are numerous breathing exercises, some thousands of years old that reportedly enhance the health and even spiritual prospects of the practitioner. For example, *kapalabhati pranayama*, a yogic practice, is used to detoxify the body, among other benefits. *Alternate nostril breathing* is said to help ground the mind, calm the practitioner and address anxiety. *Ocean breath* exercise is said to counter anger. What we know from a scientific perspective is that deep breathing (stomach breathing) has many physical and psychological benefits.

When the nervous system is adequately oxygenated, the brain, spinal cord, and nerves become more nourished and communicate more efficiently with all the other systems of the body, thereby enhancing the health of these systems. This oxygenation benefits digestive organs, helping them to function more efficiently. Stomach breathing massages the intestines, liver, stomach, lungs, heart, and pancreas and helps support them. Oxygenation strengthens the immune system and helps the body to metabolize nutriments, build muscles, and burn fat. Deep breathing brings oxygenation to all the cells of the body and releases up to seventy percent of the toxins expunged by the body, resulting in less work for the other organs involved in the process. Breathing exercises release neurochemicals into the brain that benefit our attitude, causing us to relax, lowering our blood pressure, and supporting clear thinking.

Yoga and qigong practices are my primary sources for breathing exercises. We can incorporate breathing exercises into our lives to ground us and optimize our daily activities and in support of our journey to healthy democracy.

Massage

Massage has many benefits. Stress, which is at the root of much illness, can be greatly reduced with massage. Massage relaxes muscles, reduces stress hormones, and increases serotonin and dopamine, both of which relieve depression and enhance feelings of joy. In addition, massage can help address stiffness in our joints and muscles.

Massage, from the perspective of optimizing subtle energy flow, can be used to open passageways for life force. These subtle energies that then permeate our bodies provide a higher level of connection to our greater essence and consequently rejuvenate us. The systems of the self can become more harmonized and balanced, offering the sensation of peace, even love. Many forms of massage can help with this quest. Some focus on the muscular systems (including connective tissue). Others deal with energy channels and energy bodies, focusing on acupressure points, the meridians in general, or reflexology areas. Often the various massage techniques have similar purposes. All are said to help clear blockages to subtle energy flow. They can be used separately, or as I have practiced, combined in a self-massage routine that helps permeate the body with chi.

For example, deep-tissue massage by a trained masseuse or by oneself with foam rollers and tennis balls can not only realign deeper layers of muscles and relax bands of rigid muscles, tendons, and ligaments, it also can help hydrate connective tissue. Connective tissue is believed to serve as a conduit to subtle energies, and massage allows these energies to better permeate our extracellular and intracellular fluids that surround and fill every cell in our bodies.

Acupressure massage (using hands and fingers), like acupuncture (using needles), stimulates the various acupoints throughout the body to release stagnation of subtle energy throughout our energetic system and consequently the other systems of the self. This energetic flow revitalizes our organs and optimizes our bodily systems such as digestive or cardiovascular. These points are like antennae that pick up subtle energy from our environment and direct it into meridians that relate to the systems of the body.

Reflexology also focuses on key areas, primarily on the feet and hands, to stimulate nerve areas that are believed to correspond to various systems of the body, thereby invigorating those systems. Reflexology is said to clear the body of toxins, improve the immune system, stimulate the nervous system, and help the body to heal itself.

Shiatsu massage also utilizes the hands and fingers to stimulate key points in our bodies as well as the meridians (rivers of energy). It speeds up or slows down the flow of energy to balance the systems of the self and treat the entire body to address health issues. I practiced Shiatsu techniques as a child to great benefit.

Do-in is another form of massage/exercise that I learned as a child. It is less known in the West even today, compared to the others mentioned. According to Michio Kushi (1979, 95),

> Do-In exercises aim toward our physical betterment and well-being, but they also aim far beyond the physical dimension toward the development of our mental and spiritual abilities for the achievement of true human nature as a whole, in all dimensions . . . .. Do-In can be practiced by anyone, in any place, using only a short period of time; and therefore, can easily be a part of our daily life, not requiring any special effort or placing a burden upon our daily activities . . . Do-In does not regard human beings as physical and material existences, but rather as manifestations of vibrational and spiritual movement, arising in the infinite dimension of vibration and energy in the ocean of the infinite universe.

Spinal Care

Not many health experts (outside the chiropractic profession) discuss the value of a well-aligned and hydrated spine. Through my experience of back and neck injuries, the importance of a healthy spine has personally been underscored. The spine, many theorists assert, is where subtle energy meets the physical. Through the spine, the healing power of the nervous system is distributed throughout our bodily systems (cardio, endocrine, digestive, and so on).

If we look at the vertebrae, we can see nerve passages emerging from each one that affect many systems in the body. For example, the first cervical vertebra relates to blood supply to the head, sympathetic nervous system, and pituitary gland, among other areas. If the nerves from this area are impinged upon or cut off, the results can be devastating or fatal. Each of the twenty-four vertebrae and the sacrum and coccyx relate to vital systems of the body and therefore must be cared for. It is important to pursue this care with caution, as the spine is delicate, and professionals should always oversee our care.

Medical doctors, chiropractors, and physical therapists are all recommended to lead us down the pathway to a healthy spine. Yoga, inversion, traction, qigong, do-in, physical therapy prescribed exercises, and an inflatable wobble cushion can also play a fundamental role in home care, particularly if one cannot afford assistance from medical professionals on a regular basis.

Cardio and Strength Training

There is an abundance of books, Internet sources, and fitness trainers to guide our approach to general exercise. The United States has become very conscious of fitness. But fitness is not necessarily the same as health. Very high levels of fitness, particularly for competitive purposes, can lead to bodily damage. Joints, cartilage, ligaments, even internal organs can be damaged with extreme efforts at achieving fitness. Exercising for health is about maximizing the body and its systems for longevity and daily function.

At its most fundamental level, exercise is about the circulation and distribution of life forces to optimize the creative elements throughout our body, mind, and soul. We are made up of multiple fields of energy woven together by numerous channels of life force, material and measurable as well as subtle and unmeasurable. Exercise enables these forces to saturate and empower our being.

There are many ways to approach exercise. Ancient methods such as qigong and yoga focus on building chi as well as flexibility and strength of muscles and ligaments. These have been my foundational approach to exercise, and I use them daily. In the West, we are more concerned with cardiovascular development, most particularly through interval training (also known to accelerate weight loss), jogging (also known to release noradrenaline), and walking (also known to help moderate sadness). I incorporate light levels of interval training with occasional jogging or walking and have found this approach very helpful as I've grown older. Cardiovascular exercise, of course, can strengthen our heart and expand our lung capacity and help perfuse our bodies with oxygen. These exercises, along with resistance training (e.g., calisthenics such as pushups and pullups for muscular endurance, weight training for strength and power and a testosterone boost, and isometrics that strengthen ligaments and muscles), are tools for strengthening the body and consequently the mind. I have found these valuable to include at a moderate level of intensity.

Exercising in most forms, done correctly, will tend to positively affect the other systems of the body, including hormones and the immune system, and help us generate better health and longevity. Explore the many various approaches and find what fits who you are. Remember, your body is a complex machine with many systems that need tuning. Consider approaching fitness from multiple disciplines (cross-training). But most of all do something for yourself— you'll feel better and people will pick that up from you as you pursue better relationships and a better world.

CHAPTER **10**

Eating to Center the Systems of the Self

> "For things to Change—you have to change.
> For things to get better—you have to get better."
> --Jim Rohn

THE BATTLEFIELD OF our cultural evolution lies in our hearts, minds and bodies. The foundation of our successful evolution is our physical fitness, a heart that loves freely and a mind liberated by cognition that is creative, responsible, continuously improving, and consequently acting in balance with the self and our greater essence. The fourth footing for this foundation is our diet. What we eat affects what we feel, think, and do. The proper foods lay the foundational chemistry that serves as a conduit to subtle energies. There is much debate about what we should eat. All sides have much ego, worldview, and wealth at stake. We have our lives at stake and the future of our democracy as well.

Along with oxygen and water, food sets the stage for a properly functioning cellular system—the cells that are the building blocks of our bodies. The architecture for all that we are physically (our genes) is erected (activated) by what we take into our bodies through our senses—what we see, breathe, smell, hear, feel—and what we absorb through our skin and what we taste and eat. How we respond or react, how we perceive, digest, assimilate these environmental energies into our being, in turn creates our reality. A structure built on an unsound footing cannot be counted on to stand. Food is fundamental to a healthy foundation from which to build our lives and the world we live in.

If we eat foods that offer probiotics and fiber, we empower our digestive system and our immune system. Eating sufficient minerals and cruciferous vegetables helps strengthen the liver, which in turn regulates and cleans the blood. Fruits that provide vitamin C and (according to traditional Chinese health systems) orange-colored foods such as cantaloupe, carrots, and squash strengthen the spleen. Foods high in Omega 3, antioxidants, and low in refined flour, sugar, and saturated fat strengthen the kidneys. Foods high in phytoestrogens (broccoli, beans, and many others) are necessary to maintain a healthy endocrine system. Quality proteins as well as nutrients such as vitamin C, phosphorus, calcium, and potassium are necessary for maintaining strong muscles, joints, and bones. What we eat (especially foods rich in B and E vitamins, acetyl carnitine, magnesium, and potassium) affects the biology of our nervous system, and this affects all our functions, including our very consciousness. Consequently, our food affects the biology of the world because we are shaping the world's biology for better or worse with what we think, feel, say, and do. So—what diet provides the footing for a long, happy, healthy life that in turn helps perpetuate a better world?

In Western society, the Food and Drug Administration (FDA) and the United States Department of Agriculture (USDA) are the leading authorities on a healthy diet. The USDA advocates what is called *MyPlate* as a map for healthy eating. This consists of about forty percent vegetables, ten percent fruit, thirty percent grains (mostly whole), twenty percent protein (mostly lean meats, beans, and nuts) and one to two servings of (nonfat) dairy daily. The FDA, according to Wells (2014), also approves over 70,000 food additives, from artificial ingredients (e.g., preservatives, coloring) to pesticides. The FDA doesn't specifically recommend supplements but instead recommends daily amounts of vitamins and minerals such as 1,000 IUs daily of vitamin D. Since it is difficult to get that much vitamin D through diet and an indoor lifestyle, supplementation, in a roundabout way, can be encouraged. Diet nonetheless remains the primary suggested means for obtaining proper nutriments.

The credibility of the FDA and USDA, has, however, been challenged. Numerous reputable dietary authorities such as John A. McDougall and T. Colin Campbell claim that these agencies are overwhelmingly shaped by corporate influence. What these authors suggest is that corporate lobbyists advocate for GMOs, pesticides, and meat and dairy products, and this results in the acceptance by government regulators of subpar research methods and faulty study conclusions that result in policies that benefit these industries at the expense of public health. Consequently, challenges to the USDA view of a healthy diet have gained popularity. Some challengers disagree based on their own academic and scientific research and that of others, their experience, and their cultural and spiritual (not to mention political!) beliefs.

Other writers have argued that the approval of foods such as GMOs and meats with added hormones are severely endangering the health of Americans. Jeffrey M. Smith in his international bestseller *Seeds of Deception* (2003) reported that numerous researchers and scientists have raised legitimate health concerns about such additives, only to have them fall on the deaf ears of FDA officials. Smith suggested that the FDA has ignored research that could prove damaging to GMO sales, and that the FDA may have even colluded with Monsanto (a leading developer of GMOs) to hide evidence of findings that underscore the dangers of some of their products. He suggested that there is evidence that the media have also participated in coverups.

Three primary groups appear to make up these challengers to the Western dietary establishment as reflected in the MyPlate percentages. One emphasizes a much higher animal protein intake, and another focuses on much higher plant-based food consumption, even exclusively so (vegan). A third, in-between, emphasis reflects various views on animal protein versus plant-based foods. Within these three groups we find seven major dietary philosophies.

Diets that advocate for higher animal protein:

(a) the Atkins diet
(b) the Paleo diet.

Diets that advocate for plant-based foods as an alternative to animal protein:

(c) those that emphasize green, leafy vegetables and fruits. (see Campbell 2006)
(d) those that emphasize starches. (see McDougall 2012)

Falling in between the first two:

(e) lactovegetarian diets (dairy but no meat, fish, or poultry)
(f) the Mediterranean diet
(g) the macrobiotic diet.

The Atkins diet challenges the USDA diet at its philosophical base by citing research and anecdotal claims that fat isn't the culprit for causing obesity, disease, and poor health—rather, it is sugar and other carbohydrates in conjunction with fats (although hydrogenated fats are to be avoided). Milk is also to be avoided (because of the carbohydrates), but full-fat cheeses, cream, and butter are allowed. According to this philosophy, it is the spiking of blood sugar (high and then low) that is at the root of obesity and many diseases. The Atkins diet has no limit on poultry, fish, shellfish, meat, and eggs. A vegetarian approach to this diet is possible using products such as tofu and olive oil, but this variation is largely obscured in the literature. Salads and vegetables, even some whole grains, red wine, and nuts can be incorporated as long as the net carbs (carbs minus their fiber content) are no more than 45–100 grams a day. Diet soda, black coffee, and tea can also be consumed. Nonprocessed foods are encouraged, as is taking a daily multivitamin–mineral and fatty acids.

The Paleo diet is based on what is believed to be early mankind's dietary habits (hunting and gathering) prior to agriculture. The idea is that this is our most natural and therefore healthiest mode of eating—what humans are genetically designed to eat. The Paleo diet, like Atkins, emphasizes animal protein, but unlike Atkins, the animal protein should be lean (particularly game meats and organ meats such as liver). It also avoids eggs and does not allow dairy (due to the sugar or fat content). Refined sugar is eliminated, as well as honey and maple syrup. It avoids all grains, arguing that grains are a part of the sugar spike problem at the root of the poor health that modern humans face.

Paleo sees legumes as a less healthy alternative to meats. Advocates warn that beans as a primary source of calories may prevent some absorbing of nutriments due to their phytic acid content. The oligosaccharides that they contain may also cause digestive problems for some. Soybeans in particular contain phytoestrogen that is said to mimic estrogen in the body. This can fool the body into believing that it has enough estrogen when it doesn't, resulting in the impairment of fertility in women. In men, phytoestrogen can potentially cause feminine traits such as breasts or fat deposits on the hips. Even grain like seeds (e.g., quinoa, amaranth), starchy vegetables, and salt-containing foods like olives and salted nuts are to be avoided.

Green leafy vegetables, berries and fruits are allowed in Paleo, as is moderate consumption of oils such as olive, avocado, walnut, and flaxseed, and moderate intake of diet sodas, coffee, tea, wine, beer, spirits, dried fruits, and nuts. Vitamins D, E, and C and selenium supplements are to be considered (fish oil is recommended for those who won't eat fish).

In the Atkins and Paleo diets, refined sugars and milk are essentially eliminated. Nutritional supplements are encouraged in varying degrees, as well as unprocessed foods. Animal protein is emphasized. De-emphasis on eating grains is a dominant characteristic of both, as grains are perceived to be a central cause of the health problems

Eating to Center the Systems of the Self

facing modern society. Writers from the antigrain school of thought, such as David Perlmutter, describe wheat as a foremost culprit among grains. According to Perlmutter (2013), wheat gluten can cause inflammation that leads to a variety of negative health conditions.

Conversely, writers such as John A. McDougall promote starch as the savior of human health and the natural foundational food for humankind. He cites research and anecdotal claims to support his assertions. McDougall (2012) prescribes a food plate consisting of seventy percent starch (e.g., barley, buckwheat, corn, millet, oats, rice, rye, sorghum, wheat, wild rice, beans, lentils, peas, starchy vegetables), twenty percent nonstarchy vegetables, and ten percent fruit. He also recommends lots of water, encourages whole foods, and recommends zero meat, fish, and dairy. Other foods to be avoided include sugar-sweetened cereal, cookies, cakes, white rice and flour, vegetable cooking oils, coffee, black tea, and sodas. He strongly discourages most supplements except B12 and possibly vitamin D. Moderate salt intake, nuts, and a small amount of refined sugar and natural sweeteners are allowed.

T. Colin Campbell used major research to point out that animal-based protein, particularly casein (milk protein), is the culprit behind obesity, cancer, and many other diseases. Campbell (2006) encourages eating as much fruit, vegetables (starchy and nonstarchy), beans, nuts, and whole grains as required to meet dietary needs. He warns about refined carbohydrates, added vegetable oils, and fish, and cautions avoidance of all meat, poultry, dairy, and eggs. He encourages whole foods and discourages vitamin supplements except B12 (and vitamin D for those who spend most of their time indoors).

On the other hand, contrary to Campbell and McDougall, the lactovegetarian diet allows milk, dairy, and eggs. Lactovegetarian diets can vary: some resemble the USDA recommendations minus the meat, fish, and poultry (replaced by vegetable protein sources and dairy). Others are guided by Ayurvedic principles. Ayurveda is a traditional Asian Indian healing system that is holistic in its approach and incorporates Indian traditional foods, herbs, spices, and flavors to positively affect health. Many vegetarians, including lactovegetarians, are also motivated by political and worldviews that are opposed to eating animals. Most lactovegetarians today appear to gravitate toward whole foods. Supplementation varies widely.

The macrobiotic and Mediterranean diets are both centered on eating grains (with different emphases on type and percentage). They also have varying emphases on type and amount of fruit and vegetables, and both include small amounts (but varying types) of animal protein.

The diet generally associated with macrobiotics is largely plant-based, with a de-emphasis on fruits and nonstarchy vegetables and the allowance of some white fish. The macrobiotic diet emphasizes whole grains (particularly brown rice), starchy vegetables such as squash, and beans. Locally grown foods are preferred, because foods are to be eaten according to the climate where one lives. In addition, fermented soy products such as miso, tofu, tamari, and tempeh are encouraged (nonfermented soy products are not recommended). Other foods often consumed are seaweeds (e.g., nori, wakame) and pickles made from such foods as umeboshi plums and daikon radish. Cooked foods are emphasized. Whole, organic food is a focus. Sesame oil and seeds, as well as sea salt, are key seasonings. Pungent spices like black pepper and cayenne are discouraged. A balance of yin and yang (alkaline and acidic) foods is a goal. Meat, dairy, and eggs are outside the recommended guidelines. Occasional rice wine is acceptable, but coffee and black tea, refined sugar, or refined grains of any sort are not used, nor are vitamin supplements. Certain herbal teas and remedies are encouraged.

The Mediterranean diet focus is on grains (preferably whole) and lots of cooked and fresh vegetables and fruits of all kinds. Olives and olive oil are used abundantly. Coffee is consumed. Milk is not used as a beverage. Cheese (particularly goat) and meat are used more as flavoring, and seafood and red wine are consumed in moderation. A small amount of refined sugar is permissible. Vitamin supplements are not typically seen as necessary.

All the above dietary approaches tend to conclude that herbal and vitamin supplements are not to be considered as replacement for food, and that food is the first line of medicine. But most of them also acknowledge that supplements can be looked on as gap fillers when our lifestyle and diet prevent us from getting some vital nutriments. I believe that supplements can also be seen as a medicine. Modern life is not an easy game to play. In interacting with our environment, we may find many toxic chemicals; we may experience stress, injury, and illnesses; and sometimes just plain old age—all can severely weaken us. Supplements, wisely used, can help. For example, fish oil can be used to reduce inflammation. St. John's wort can help to relieve depression. Coenzyme Q10 and calcium have been shown to reduce hypertension. It takes wisdom and study to know which supplements to take and how to take them. But it is worth taking the time to ascertain how herbal and nutritional supplements may help you meet your particular needs. A nutritionist and herbalist should be used as a guide to supplements.

What all the diets above absolutely have in common are the claims of some degree of tradition, as well as science and anecdotal evidence, to support each in its assertion that its respective dietary approach produces leaner physiques and, more importantly, healthier, longer, and happier lives. Yet these dietary approaches often appear to totally contradict each other. So which one is the correct diet?

One school of thought is that it isn't what we eat but the nutriments (including micronutrients) we get from our food and their synergy that are most important. Although the regions of the world with the longest-living people tend to consume plant-based diets that include grains or starchy vegetables and a small amount of animal protein, people from all over the world have achieved good health within a range of greatly divergent diets—some consisting almost entirely of animal protein and fat and others of almost all plant-based foods. In all cases, however, the foods eaten are largely unprocessed and are local, naturally raised, or wild. Others suggest that what is most healthy to eat depends on our individual genetics, our current environment (stress levels, pollution), our current health, age, and even climate. According to Gary L. Wenk (2010), diet is as much about the *quantity* of what we eat as it is about what foods we eat: "Because we consume food, we must consume oxygen. Because we consume oxygen, we age. Thus, people who live the longest tend to eat foods rich in antioxidants or simply eat much less food."

The dietary habits of those residing in areas with the longest-living inhabitants on Earth support this claim, as does much research. Perhaps, as the Okinawan saying goes, we should "only eat when we're hungry and only eat till we're eighty percent full." It's likely that eating light and getting the right nutriments from natural unprocessed foods will contribute to longer, happier, healthier lives. It seems sensible to avoid eating foods high in sugar (particularly refined) and low in fiber, as these practices tend to be largely discouraged by all the dietary schools of thought reviewed. All the above diets, to varying degrees, encourage nonstarchy vegetables. Dairy products, particularly cow's milk, may be for many of us something to consider reducing or eliminating altogether. Most of the USDA challengers steer away from drinking milk, although sometimes for different reasons. Additionally, a close look at the impact that wheat gluten may have on one's health may be worthwhile.

What most of these diets have in common is the tendency to produce an alkaline chemistry in the body as opposed to an acidic one (with the exceptions of the Atkins diet, as well as the traditional American diet with lots of refined sugar, white flour, and fewer fruits and vegetables). Acidic body chemistry can lead to inflammation. Inflammation is believed by many (both mainstream and holistic health experts) to be an underlying cause for many diseases. Foods that produce an acidic condition in the body include saturated fats, meats, poultry, fish, dairy (except perhaps buttermilk), coffee, black tea, alcohol, refined sugar, and flours. Foods that produce an alkaline condition include many vegetables; some fruits like bananas, limes, and watermelon; some beans such as lima beans; nuts such as almonds; cayenne peppers; and olive oil, among many others.

Balancing acidic foods with alkaline foods may be key for achieving optimal health.

The balance of pH is measured on a scale of 0 – 14 with 7 being neutral, zero being extreme acidic and 14 extremely alkaline. According to nutritionist Millie Lytle, ND (2013), for optimal health, the body maintains a pH balance of 7. 4. Below 7.4 the blood is too acidic and when the pH is above 7.4 the blood is too alkaline. The body uses buffer systems, exhalation, and the elimination of hydrogen ions through the kidneys as mechanisms to maintain pH balance. However, if our diets are extremely imbalanced (too acidic or alkaline), this can cause these mechanisms to break down and weaken over time. The consequence is that we can become too acidic or too alkaline. This imbalance is a precursor to many diseases.

Our pH balance is measured in the fluids in our bodies—specifically, the intracellular fluid in all the cells of the body and extracellular fluid consisting of plasma and interstitial fluid that fills the spaces around the tissues of the body. According to Cyndi Dale (2009, 172), connective tissue theory is

> based on the existence of cytoskeletal structures in every cell in the body. These structures, in effect, form connective tissue. Nuclear magnetic resonance has shown that the muscles are organized in a "liquid-crystalline-like" structures that change drastically when exposed to electromagnetic fields. This alteration occurs because connective tissue carries static electric charges and is influenced by pH, salt concentrations, and the dielectric constant of the solvent. Many scientists now believe that the meridians lie within this "liquid network," or at least, stimulate its responsiveness. In other words, this liquid network carries the electromagnetic responses elicited from acupuncture.

What we eat may help create the proper pH balance in our bodily fluids to optimally conduct subtle energy. On the other hand, if our diet is too acidic or alkaline producing, it can create a pH balance that can serve as a poor conductor of subtle energy, causing our systems to degenerate and fail. A balanced diet, theoretically, brings the self in better balance with our greater essence because it is better able to attract and conduct chi in order to empower the systems of the self.

The prescription for each of us with respect to diet remains elusive, because only experiencing our own bodies can tell us what exactly is the best diet for us. Each of us must build our own food plate customized to our specific state of health, genetics, age, and environment. We must all set forth on an adventure to discover what makes us honestly feel and perform our best. Whole, nonprocessed foods are preferred overall by the above diets (even the USDA MyPlate), and I also encourage certified organic, as it is the surest way to avoid GMO and pesticide treated foods (I say this for political reasons as well). By committing to whole, organic foods, we commit to realizing our connection to the natural world. In addition, eating light is a very good place to start for building a food plate customized for the life we want to live.

Experiment. Start with green nonstarchy vegetables and build around them with local, seasonal fruits or starchy vegetables high in antioxidants. Investigate nightshade vegetables (potatoes, peppers, eggplant), as some holistic medicine traditions such as homeopathy claim these can cause inflammation. Then add in a variety of other foods that are high in antioxidants such as berries, oranges, pomegranates, peppers, spinach, cabbage, red beans, pinto beans, corn, and oats. Include other grains such as rice, barely, millet, quinoa and rye. As to animal protein, besides the health reasons, there is of course much political motivation for not eating it (environmental impact, animal rights).

If you decide to eat meat or dairy, I encourage you to keep to the natural theme by consuming grass-fed, organic meats and dairy; wild-caught fish and organic eggs; and nonantibiotic-raised poultry. Add various spices as time goes on. Finally, wine or beer, coffee, and teas can be added. If, as you expand your diet, you notice physical/

emotional/mental or even spiritual setbacks, these may be signs that the foods you are consuming are negatively affecting you, and you may want to rethink including them in your diet. Finally, all dietary approaches would agree to stay well hydrated.

If money is an issue, consider organic frozen vegetables. They are often much cheaper and just as nutritious. Research and discover which foods should be the priority in terms of which are less affected by pesticides. Livestrong.com (March 2017), listed nineteen foods to always buy organic (meat, dairy, apples, blueberries, celery, cherry tomatoes, cucumbers, grapes, corn, hot peppers, leafy greens, nectarines, peaches, potatoes, snap peas, soy, spinach, strawberries, sweet bell peppers.) The same article listed sixteen that have less pesticide residue (onions, avocado, pineapple, asparagus, grapefruit, mangoes, kiwi fruit, mushrooms, papaya, sweet peas, cantaloupe, sweet potatoes, eggplant, cabbage, watermelon, and cauliflower). It is important to note that some of these items can be GMO, such as papaya, and that should also be a consideration.

Keep a journal of what you eat and how you feel as you experiment. Be honest with yourself about how the foods you eat make you feel and perform, because your life and the life of this world could depend on it. Remember, energy follows consciousness, and the focus of our consciousness creates reality. If we focus on consuming food as a diversion from our greater purpose (long, happy, healthy lives that contribute to a better world), we are defeating our purpose for eating, and we could be contributing to a dark reality that we might end up living in.

If as a society our focus for producing food is on profit, even at the expense of health, then food developed with this focus will follow suit. The products that result will beg to be made addictive. Historically, some of the most corrupted among us, such as cult leaders, pimps, and pushers, have used addiction as a tool of control. So it is with the food production/marketing/distribution system of our modern society. Our consciousness has been redirected to focus in a manner that has addicted us to food products that are killing us.

We are manipulated to surrender our health (our bodies) and our environment so others can build greater and greater wealth and power over us. These addictions serve as barriers between us and a more disciplined focus on building a freer life through health. Health allows us to be and do more of the things we *will* to be and do. Addiction enslaves us and robs us of our free will.

The more we participate in a system that promotes eating GMOs and 70,000 different chemical additives and pesticides, the more we become a part of the antilife that it represents and the expansion of the darkness that it pursues. We merge our energies with death—we accelerate our dying physically, mentally, emotionally, and spiritually. We spread antilife into our families, communities, and nations. To fully free ourselves from the Few, we must free ourselves from addictive behaviors that are destructive to our health, lives, and relationships, and this includes what foods we choose to eat and why we choose to eat them.

Although many things can be addictive, just about any addictive substance, even those with well-known devastating consequences, can sometimes be used constructively. So we must be *conscious* of the reasons why we eat what we eat as well as the impact on our health and vitality. These reasons will affect our overall quality of life and the world. Is your diet helping you to create a long, happy, healthy life that contributes to a better world? What reality are you pursuing when it comes to eating?

I will conclude by saying that a holistic approach to wellness offers many benefits. Wellness has changed my life. It was wellness that refocused my direction from one of certain chaos and destruction to one that created a happy, healthy, constructive way of being. I have lived a life of contribution to my community and love and responsibility to my family. Wellness practices have helped me to improve my health as well as manage my anger and enable the dissolution of my violent behavior.

To be clear, I am not suggesting that wellness practices are a cure-all and be-all to our lives. No matter how well we become, we will always be human, with all the frailties and faults associated with the human condition. I believe balance is very important in achieving wellness—both in respect to fitness and in a curative sense. I think it is also important to note that there are many claims that holistic health practices can cure numerous ailments that Western medicine cannot currently cure. Some of this may be true; however, it is also true that, for a variety of reasons, research in support of such claims is lacking.

In my experience with wellness practices, they are first and foremost complementary and preventive in application and are rarely a total replacement for modern Western medicine. Using such methods, in my experience is usually beneficial at the predisease or early stages of ailments such as prehypertension and diabetes. There is some evidence that diet and healing practices such as qigong have healed certain advanced ailments that Western medicine has deemed incurable, but most of this evidence is anecdotal, and more research is needed.

Western medicine is profit driven and symptomatic treatment of disease, and this has its limitations. Nonetheless, Western medicine saves countless lives every year. In contrast, the theories behind holistic and traditional medical practices focus on the cause of disease. Because of the success of wellness approaches and holistic healthcare, these practices are showing up more in the scientific literature, and it is becoming harder for the scientific community to ignore their value in improving health. Consequently, more and more Western medical practitioners are taking an integrated approach, using both holistic and traditional Western medicine to optimize healing and promote wellness in general.

Holistic wellness is important to healthy democracy because our behavior and consequently our relationships are built on our emotional, mental, and physical wellness. Democracy reflects the people who it serves. If we want a healthy democracy, we must also strive for a healthy populace. It would be of great benefit to the democracy movement if the leaders of the most successful local grassroots social betterment organizations (right and left) convened from across the nation annually to explore wellness practices. Not only would it infuse the grassroots with a greater consciousness of wellness, but provide an important networking environment.

I'm not saying that in order to have a healthy democracy, we must all eat granola and chant (unless that is what works for you). What I'm saying is that there are abundant approaches to consider with respect to eating and exercising our way to wellness. I'm also saying that the journey to wellness is imperative for each of us to undertake for the sake of our lives, our families and our nation, because our nation is a reflection of our bodies, hearts and minds.

CHAPTER **11**

You Are the DNA of Democracy

> Be the change you want to see in the world.
> —Gandhi

FROM THE VERY beginning of my life, I found myself confronted by issues that centered on human diversity—diversity of races, regions, religions, gender, spirituality, politics, class, and culture. I was compelled to think about many of these issues, even as a small child. Learning to swim in this rough and tumultuous sea of conflicting values and norms was a matter of survival. It shaped me—made me who I am today. As a youth on the brink of manhood, I found myself grappling to address the issues posed by diversity, and this struggle became a lifelong quest for answers. I found myself involved in organizational effort after organizational effort—each on the cutting edge of addressing the enigma of bringing together diversity (essentially conflict, often right vs. right) in order to create harmony and effectiveness in organizations and communities. Eventually, this experience led me to academia for answers, where I studied grassroots groups and other organizations that strived to involve the diversity of people they served in shaping their works. In the DNA of these organizational processes and structures, the meaning of healthy democracy became clear.

What I found was that healthy democracy exists, in its most fundamental form, in how we relate to each other as human beings. *Very* simplistically speaking, *healthy democracy* is a structured balance between the mentalities of "I, me, mine" and "us, we, ours"—a balance between individualism and mutualism. A healthy democracy involves constituent representation and direct constituent participation through a governing order that is *focused on the expressed requirements of the constituents*, innovative, effectively and efficiently managed, and based fundamentally on the rules akin to the value that is common among the major religions of the world—what Christians know as the *Golden Rule*. Through these characteristics, democracy becomes an authentic governing process of, by, and for all the people equitably.

The process of healthy democracy starts with the individual and is extended through relationships: first with family, friends, neighbors, and community members, and then local, state, national, and international government representatives. But the revelation is in the focus and structural details of the effective, efficient, and Golden Rule aspects as well as the style with which the representatives and leaders serve. These characteristics elucidate why healthy democracy offers hope in addressing the issues posed by our cultural diversity. These characteristics make clear why healthy democracy is the natural counter to the colonization of humanity promoted by those who have mastered setting that diversity against itself to selfishly, and ruthlessly, exploit the resources of the world.

Through understanding what constitutes healthy democracy from an organizational behavior perspective, we can see the underlying evolutionary and spiritual nature of our journey as human beings. Through healthy democracy, individuals pursue their own needs while also focusing on the Golden Rule—and in so doing strive to create a society that promises to uphold humanities highest ideals for society—a more reciprocal–altruistic culture for all of humanity.

Power is control of energy. If energy follows consciousness, then control of reality is power. Those who control reality control humanity. Those who control their own consciousness control their own reality. Personal power begins with self-control. Leadership for a healthy democracy begins with our ability to shape our own destiny without losing sight of empathy for others—connecting us, inspiring each other, and transforming our world to serve the needs of all the people through mutuality.

We all have a sphere of influence. For a few of us this sphere is very great, perhaps an entire nation. For others it may be limited to our own behavior. What matters is not how large our sphere of influence is, but what we do within our sphere of influence to change the world that is the measure of one's contributions to our cultural evolution.

According to Martin Lindstrom (2008), we are all neurologically predisposed to be influenced by environmental stimuli such as memes. Lindstrom described mirror neurons as powerful biological bases for much of humanity's behavior. Mirror neurons encourage us to reflect the behavior of others around us. Our reflective nature suggests that we have the potential to reflect cultural values, norms, and cultural artifacts established not only by formal leadership, but also, and perhaps more importantly, by informal leadership. Let your behavior be a light for others to reflect!

Christakis and Fowler in their book *Connected* (2009) suggested that both our behavior and our emotions can impact individuals three times removed from us—that is, our friend's, friend's friend. By being what you espouse, you can establish a form of leadership. By treating others in the manner you feel should be the norm of humanity, you can be influential. I would argue that if you afford liberty, you build the case for your own liberty. If you authentically engage in charity, you strengthen the case for advocating greater charity in society. Ultimately, how you act in your circle of influence will be your greatest power for influencing others within that circle and perhaps, in turn, the circles of those you influence. Your behavior can affect the behavior of others. This is the essence of leadership.

The leadership for healthy democracy is not leadership from above at all, but leadership from below—a leadership rooted in empathy: "The poor serving the poor," as Saint Theresa of Calcutta would say. This leadership arises out of common experiences. It is focused on addressing the needs of others. This service is guided by empathetic relationships that provide the motivation to pursue the requirements of those in need.

The authentic leaders for healthy democracy do not stand above those in need; they stand with them and among them. They are not so much the visionaries as the facilitators of vision that emerges from the people. Leadership from above is at best divided leadership: the servant of two masters. The very essence of being anointed by the established system of power indicates support for policy and process that maintains the dominance of the power elite. Acceptance from the power elite requires a lack of authentic demand for fundamental change on the part of the leaders who are positioned to lead from above—that is, to manage the status quo. What I mean is that any leadership sanctioned by a system of the status quo (e.g., governments, business sector, major media, mainstream academia, political parties) is unlikely to be an agent of fundamental change, much less an agent for a healthy democracy. Leaders tend to serve best those whom they relate to. When leaders are themselves a part of the elite, they will tend to serve the elite best of all, as they not only have intimate knowledge of their needs and desires, but will also likely have a heartfelt connection with their positions and therefore personal motivation to serve those positions.

The status quo is threatened by fundamental change driven by leadership from below. Perhaps that is why it is questionable whether a healthy democracy truly represented by the people, rooted in a human rights ethic akin to the Golden Rule, has fully evolved alongside our technological advancements. It appears likely that each major nation in the world today, to varying degrees, is still driven by the political and economic elite—and the elite by their very nature would not sanction their own demise. Consequently, our technological advancement tends to serve the needs of the powerful, not democracy. Therefore, leadership from below must lead this evolution of human culture. The leadership of everyday men, women, and children is what is required. Only leadership from below can transform the leadership style of this nation. Only leadership from below can guide a macrocultural evolution of humankind that is more oriented toward the masses. By becoming a leader in this respect, we begin to take control of the third pillar of power—control of leadership.

To contribute leadership to macrocultural change along the lines of healthy democracy, one thing we can do is to clarify our own lives. This clarification can be used to support being a change agent for healthy democracy in our professional as well as our personal lives. This doesn't mean you must wait until you are perfect to participate in creating healthy democracy and environments that breed healthy democracy—no! Rather, we must understand who we are and where we are in our lives as we proceed down this vital path toward contributing to human cultural evolution as well as our own.

In their reference to nonprofit organizations, Minkoff and Powell (in Powell and Steinberg 2006, 591) described a mission as "a clarion call." *Collins* online dictionary defines *clarion call* as "a strong emotional appeal to people to do something." In the context of a personal life mission, this means that your mission statement must be deeply meaningful to yourself and that it must inspire action based on deep, core values. It does not matter if others find your mission statement attractive or meaningful. What matters is that your life mission sums up what *you feel and think* is most important to achieve in your life, and that it encourages the pursuit of those ends.

Dr. Stephen R. Covey offers an approach for clarifying our purpose in life in his books *How to Develop Your Personal Mission Statement* (2013) and *How to Develop Your Family Mission Statement* (2012). Covey suggests that not only individuals but also families can clarify their lifelong mission. Covey's process is straightforward. In short, you reflect on the purpose for living—the purpose of *your* life. After all is said and done, what is it that you would like to accomplish during your time on Earth? Beginning with the outcome you desire for your life, what is it that you would most like to achieve? Reflect and take notes on your thoughts. Take your time.

When you think that you are close to ascertaining your mission, write down various drafts of your mission statement. Keep it as short and direct as possible, preferably a line or two. Think of your mission statement as an open-ended goal that you will pursue throughout your life. Do not include how you will pursue that goal—describe only the goal. That goal should feel to you like a call to action. Again, it does not matter if anyone else relates to it or not. This mission is for you, so don't rush the process, and make sure it is authentic. Once you have written the statement, you then can develop objectives that will guide your daily activities. Covey suggests five areas of objectives: material, physical, emotional, intellectual, and spiritual.

Below I have included my mission statement as an example. It is not a particularly heroic mission statement, but it does not have to be. What is important is that the mission is meaningful to *me*. It is a clarion call to pursue what is most important to me.

My life mission is to *enjoy life to its fullest and help create a better world*. Neither enjoying my life to its fullest nor helping to create a better world shall impede the other. In pursuit of this mission, the following life objectives will steer my daily activities.

Material Objectives: Maximize my economic independence; live a prosperous life; enjoy a comfortable retirement; provide for my family's education; and support worthy causes.

Physical Objectives: Maximize control of my time and physical location; be proficient at qigong; maintain balanced body chemistry, internal health, physical fitness, and abundant energy for work, service, and play.

Emotional Objectives: Be at peace with my life. Be the best father I can be—the kind of person I hope that any child would want to emulate or associate with. Be a true friend and sensitive partner to my wife for life. Celebrate every opportunity with my family. Enjoy social opportunities with friends and acquaintances. Empathize with others.

Intellectual Objectives: *Respond* to my internal and external environments instead of *reacting*. Take a *plan, do, check, and act* approach to life. Be a lifelong learner. Be a competent teacher. Keep an open mind.

Spiritual Objectives: Listen to the inner voice of intuition—the light and the way—my higher self (the Christ within). Continuously realize my connection to all things. Treat and think about others the way I want to be treated and thought about and how I want my loved ones to be treated and thought about. Pray.

Your life mission statement and goals may be totally different from mine, exactly like them, or someplace in between. What matters is that the statements represent *your* deepest values for *your* life. If we pursue our life's mission that evidences a value for healthy democracy, we join forces with the democratization that is awakening the world over.

Once you are clear with your own life mission, then it may be easier for you to be a light for change around you. There is no greater place to start shining the light that you find on your journey to betterment than on your family. We weave the fabric of society at home. To the extent that the Few and those who cooperate with them have control of the family, they have control of humanity. There is no more important arena for human cultural evolution than the family structure. Approaching family members with empathy opens our heart's reservoir, and by so doing we help to fill the veins of society with our greater essence—love. Using Covey's methods, we can develop family mission statements that can be used to help us focus our continuous improvement efforts. Whenever we fall off track, we can come back to our mission, evaluate our failed efforts, and improve our next attempt at pursuing our mission. By together developing a family mission statement, we take the first step to controlling the organization of society. Control of organization is the fourth pillar of power.

In our commitment to family mission statements, we can see the anchors of healthy democracy emerge—a process that is people focused, based on empathetic relationships committed to continuous improvement, and stabilized through cultural artifacts (such as mission statements) that document and perpetuate our highest values.

The following is my family mission statement as an example. I interviewed my family members and worked and reflected with them to identify the objectives important in achieving our family mission for several months before I drafted the statement.

Our family mission is to belong, love, enjoy, support, and safeguard (B.L.E.S.S.) each other as we journey through life.

Belonging: Our family strives to always offer each other a sense of belonging, a trustworthy community to connect with.

Love: Our family strives to love each other with all our hearts. This means we commit our best efforts to offer each other a heart filled with so much love that there is no room for resentment, anger, greed, or envy.

Enjoyment: Our family strives to enjoy our time together throughout our lives. We strive to take every opportunity to recreate together. We seek to savor and share simple pleasures as well as major adventures that life offers.

Support: Our family strives to support each other's best interest with all our intent. We are committed to offering each other words, thoughts, and deeds that maximize each other's best potential through the ups and downs of life.

Safeguard: Our family is committed to preventing individuals or circumstances from undermining the above commitments.

Creating a family statement is a great way to begin the practice of creating healthy democracy. It is a participatory process reliant on empathy and individual initiative. Moreover, pursuing the family mission statement is the practice of balancing the mentalities of "I, me, mine" and "us, we, ours." Through working to strengthen our families, we are weaving the fabric of society with the values that create our nation. This doesn't mean, of course, that I'm asking you to give your children the same decision-making authority as you and your spouse or partner. Rather, when we are truly family-focused, the requirements of all members, particularly children, are better understood and more likely addressed. This helps us understand what it means to have a citizen-focused society—and that is what a healthy democracy assures.

Another approach that may be helpful in preparing oneself for the journey to promoting a healthy democracy is the technique of Frederic M. Hudson (2001, 54). The adult human development theory developed by the Hudson institute described a four-phase cycle that humans go through approximately every decade.

> Phase I: Going For It, striving for your dream, and plateauing.
> Phase II: The Doldrums, i.e., the thrill is gone and change is required, which either results in a minitransition or an ending phase/letting go.
> Phase III: Cocooning, a healing and rebuilding stage.
> Phase IV: Getting Ready, i.e., exploring, preparing to launch again into the going-for-it phase.

According to The Hudson Institute of Santa Barbara "Planning for Change" workbook (2000, 8-12, abridged), for each of these phases, there are skills that Hudson helps the practitioners of his process to develop.

> Phase I skills: Dreaming/visioning, planning and pursuing goals; plateauing, and evaluating.
> Phase II skills: Managing the doldrums, sorting things out; letting go or restructuring.
> Phase III skills: Healing, introspection, reflection, recovery, and sustained resilience.
> Phase IV skills: Experimenting, networking, training/learning, being creative.

The goal of Hudson's work is to help individuals be aware of the ebb and flow of life. His work provides guidance in how to navigate through the various phases and how to respond to these phases rather than reacting to various themes that life presents. I see the process as selecting the future as opposed to surrendering to the will of others or events. The process promotes self-empowerment over passivity, and this is part of the process of healthy democracy.

Once we find that we are in the launching life cycle (and are clear about our life's mission), we're more prepared to serve as change agents or innovators within organizations that we are involved with or in the creation of new organizations or ventures. If we are better oriented in regard to our life cycle, we will be better prepared to help strengthen cooperatives, participate in community gardens, or create more participative programming in the social service or social action programs that we are involved in. Perhaps we will choose to help encourage greater social responsibility or community involvement in our place of work or even help create worker unions, encourage local empowerment efforts, engage in advocacy for more polling places, or help get out the vote.

Parents, in particular, can shape our future, not only through the development of their children, but by helping to shape our educational process through participating in PTOs, lobbying, or running for school boards on a platform of comprehensive democracy and social and emotional learning (SEL) K–12 curricula. Today Americans are largely functionally illiterate with regard to democracy. Students K–12 should be steeped in democratic ideology and practice designed appropriately for every grade level. Not only should they understand how laws are made so they can follow the development of bills and advocate effectively, they should understand the strengths, weaknesses, and threats to democracy. They should have a deep and debate-sourced understanding of the Constitution, the Bill of Rights, and the Federalist Papers that outlined the concerns of our founding fathers for protecting and furthering American democracy. All students should be well versed in discourse ethics, democratic processes, and the many forms and shapes of democracy. All American youth should graduate from high school with a profound understanding of the theory and practice of democracy through study and hands-on experiences. This preparation for participation in the democratic process, along with K–12 social and emotional learning designed to support not only student academic achievement but also the achievement of a more efficient democracy, would be evolutionary. According to research (see Jones, S. et al, 2017), SEL (Social and Emotional Learning) helps to develop self-awareness, self-management, empathy, perspective-taking, conflict resolution, and cooperation. Democracy and social and emotional learning should be core studies on par with math and science. Comprehensive SEL along with civics and democracy training in every K–12 school throughout our nation alone would revolutionize the evolution of our democracy in one generation!

As more of us move toward influencing organizations in the direction of becoming democratic, I recommend that those of us engaged in this organizational change consider ourselves to be leaders—at least of our own lives—in a cultural evolutionary process geared toward the success of humanity. In pursuit of this goal, I encourage the development, in the context of this work, of several personal characteristics:

1. the will and fortitude to set aside ego
2. the ability to be centered emotionally, intellectually, and spiritually in the collective image of the common good
3. the courage to serve the common good
4. as the primary path, the wisdom to acknowledge the experience of the group without disregarding the knowledge of the individual
5. respect for the process of compromise
6. skills in the way of collaboration
7. an ability to transform conflict into harmony
8. knowledge that diverse and even conflicting truths can coexist in a state of respect

9. wisdom to see setbacks as opportunities for growth
10. a commitment to continuous self-improvement
11. the ability to research and act, as well as to evaluate for utilization
12. the ability to respond to the environment instead of simply reacting to it
13. a commitment to practicing empathy
14. cultivate intuition.

These are the things that have been helpful for me. As I reflect on my own experiences with leadership, I realize that I've made some of my best decisions when I have *not* been able to empirically determine the definitive answer and have had to feel my way through issues of leadership. Sensing my way through conflict has helped me understand consensus as dynamic and changing—a moving forward by creating acts of collectively defined justice. I've learned that leadership isn't always inspiring others to do what you need them to do; sometimes it is about others inspiring you to do what they need *you* to do. This epiphany did not come easily to me.

I've also learned to incorporate into the leadership process more of my own human nature—not only intellectual faculties, but also my assets—physical, emotional, and spiritual. Perhaps what I'm describing when I say *spiritual* is some sort of creativity-based or intuitive leadership. Whatever it is, I believe it is an important piece of the foundation for leading collaborations comprising diverse members. I see the experience as spiritual because it helps me realize my connection to the whole of the universe, including all of humankind. This sense of leadership seeks to bring together humanity as a family. Therefore, it prescribes the value that all the great religions have in common.

I believe that we human beings are biological entities—physical, intellectual, emotional, and cultural (memes). I also believe we are spiritual beings. What a spiritual being is specifically, I have no way of empirically knowing. Perhaps cause and effect extends infinitely, but at this moment we cannot measure either the fullness of effect or the deepest origin of cause. Such a reality would make us infinite. I believe the seen and the unseen coexist. Perhaps God and Satan, good and evil, play out their never-ending antagonism in our genes and memes. But I believe that the genes and memes reflect a greater existence that transcends our physical senses and intellectual capacity.

I believe that when we lead, we deal with the sum of this soup of physical, intellectual, emotional, cultural, and spiritual existence. We draw on all these facets of ourselves to do the work required of leadership committed to bringing greater constructive interaction among human diversity and ultimately the vast diversity of life here on Earth. In this soup, boundaries are often unclear, conflicting, and ever-changing, and so leadership must be like water seeking equilibrium. Part of this equilibrium is owning-up to the fact that a commitment to healthy democracy reflects a set of values and therefore reflects a particular worldview. The leadership must be honest enough to admit that it is not altogether above bias. Without this admission, leadership will nurture the hypocrisy that is the seed of failure of such efforts.

The late Dr. Robert Terry, a respected authority on the subject of leadership, asserted that true "leadership is the courage to bring forth, and let come forth, authentic action in common." This description is especially important for people who act as leaders in collaborative efforts marked by a commitment to human diversity through the process of healthy democracy. However, it is important to add that leadership for the many includes the courage to *not* bring forth and to *not let* come forth authentic-action in common as well. I say this in reference to the presocial mind attributes inherent in us all.

There can be authentic action that comes from within us, within our groups and the collaborations that we are involved in, where coexistence with the values underlying the commitment to justly serve the many is not an option. There will be opportunities for our own group (e.g., class, political party, ethnicity, religion) to benefit by gaining what we need and feel we deserve at the expense of others by directly or indirectly infringing on their rights and even their human dignity. In such cases, leaders are faced with competing values. They are forced to support one at the expense of the other. The question that confronts us is this: is this leadership required to transcend group loyalty to serve the broader, more inclusive values posed by the spirit of supporting a more reciprocal–altruistic world—a healthy democracy?

This is a matter of credibility. Leaders will fall on a continuum of credibility depending on how they answer this question. A resounding "yes" would be the highest level of credibility, and an absolute "no" would be at the lowest. The greater the diversity that the leader serves, the higher they must score on this scale of credibility, but all must be able to accept this ultimate responsibility to effectively participate in a healthy democracy. Without credibility in this regard, there is no leadership for healthy democracy. To be consistent with the values that form the premise for healthy democracy, leadership must have the courage, at times, to stand up against actions that are authentic and justified to those individuals who perpetuate them when their actions infringe on acts of collectively defined justice, the dignity of the vulnerable, and the greater common good. Leaders of healthy democracy must be prepared to pursue effective, efficient solutions of the people, by the people, and for all the people equitably. Leadership that lacks this courage fails to support the underlying ideas and values of healthy democracy; consequently, their credibility is lost to hypocrisy.

The actions of leaders committed to healthy democracy, by definition, are interacting with a variety of views and values. To constructively engage these views and values, leaders must hold firmly to the common goal (mission/constitution/bill of rights—the Golden Rule!) while encouraging acts of collectively defined justice. They must foster respect for self-determination among the individuals but not at the expense of self-determination of the many striving toward the common good. We must create safeguards for equity of minority groups, but not diminish equity for majority classes. We must move forward with the will of the many, but not disregard the needs of the minority. With these guiding principles, leadership must be prepared to constructively engage those seeking to fulfill their needs at the expense of others with respect if even only the faintest opportunity for bridge-building exists. We must be able to forgive while not allowing ourselves to be abused. We must never forget Dawkins' Suckers, Grudgers, and Cheats! Our leaders must pursue reciprocity, because without it, our long-term evolutionary fate promises to be bleak.

The responsibility of leadership in support of healthy democracy lies with every individual who holds strongly to this value. This leadership is the voice deep within the soul of all humanity, be it gene or meme, God, or transcendent natural order. It compels us to set aside our greed, but not our need; to set aside our ethnocentricity, but not our survival; to set aside our fear in order to know empathy; and to set aside our hatred long enough to experience agape love.

CHAPTER **12**

Formally Organizing Humanity for Healthy Democracy

> "Never doubt that a small group of thoughtful, committed, citizens can change the world. Indeed, it is the only thing that ever has."
> —Margaret Mead

WE HAVE SEEN that power is control of reality, because energy follows consciousness. By focusing our consciousness on holistic wellness, we can become more effective participants in our lives and in the creation of healthy democracy. We have explored how to approach the four pillars of power—the control of economics, control of information, control of leadership, and control of organization informally, within our personal lives. Control of these pillars of power within our personal lives focuses our consciousness on creating reality based on *our* requirements. John Kenneth Galbraith (1983) in his seminal work *The Anatomy of Power* described three sources of power:

1. personality (leadership and charisma)
2. property (wealth and money)
3. organization.

Of these three sources of power organization is the most important. It is organization that magnifies the first two sources of power. We will now explore the characteristics of healthy democracy in the context of organizational behavior and how these characteristics can help structure a healthy democratic reality within our grassroots organizations and communities, and ultimately, our nation and perhaps the world.

The Formal Organization

We human beings have come to dominate the Earth because we have been able to shape our environment through organization. We are genetically responsive to our environment. These genetic responses include (to widely varying degrees, of course) both genocidal reactions toward others in our environment as well as Christ like responses. We must now organize our own evolution by creating a society that shapes the environment of humankind so that it elicits the latter response. With control of the formal organization, it is possible to distribute information that we require to free us and that *we* determine is most useful to us. Through control of formal organization, we can structure our economies to benefit the many and develop leadership to serve the needs of the people. Through the control of formal organization, the many can potentially create an environment that encourages genetic expressions latent within the population that are more reciprocal and altruistic in nature and encourage more Christ like responses toward each other and all life on Earth.

According to Robbins (1998, 2), an organization is "a consciously coordinated social unit, composed of two or more people, that functions on a relatively continuous basis to achieve a common goal or set of goals." Our organizations have emerged in response to our environment. These organizations have essentially created subenvironments that shape us (socialize us) and prepare us to meet the challenges of the external world. Through families and clans, to militaries, nations, and multinational corporate empires, humanity has risen from the dust of the Earth to dominate the globe through organizations that shape us. Consequently, humanity's success at organizing may have also brought our species to a crucial fork in the road of evolution. Can our ability to organize save us from an Orwellian future? Can our organizations help us to circumvent world crisis? Can humanity organize for healthy democracy?

To answer these questions, we explored characteristics of ourselves that drive our direction as human beings and consequently the organizations that we animate. What drives us to pursue goals that risk the rise of totalitarianism, global warming, and nuclear war? More importantly, what innate qualities in humankind could move us toward successfully organizing for justice and a healthier, more peaceful world? The quest to answer these questions led us to examine our evolutionary foundations. The answers to the above questions are found not only in our genes and memes, but also in the human environment and the ultimate impact this environment could have on the biology of human behavior. The ultimate solution to the problem humanity now faces—that is, a world dominated by totalitarians threatening war and environmental destruction—could be wrapped up in the interplay of our biology and human cultural evolution reflected in our social structures that shape us (the environments we create): our families, social networks, organizations, economies and governments.

Dawkins (1989) believes that past preprogrammed survival strategies influence contemporary human behavior. According to Dawkins, in antiquity, survival was a matter of eat or be eaten. Greed, ruthless lust, and violence were helpful in perpetuating genes and in surviving in a hostile environment. Looking out for number one comes naturally; too much sharing might distract from the human prime objective. Nonetheless, Dawkins asserted that as humanity developed more evolved social units, some instincts had to be modified. As society developed, so has human capability to affect the environment of the world.

Today, humanity's greatest challenge to survival is humanity itself. Collaboration, or at least cooperation, is becoming more and more important for our mutual survival worldwide. Global warming, by definition shared by the world, is largely the fault of several industrialized and emerging industrialized nations; their cooperation is vital to solving this problem. The drive for economic growth threatens the world's environments; world cooperation is needed to manage this growth as well. Human technologies capable of the total annihilation of life on Earth loom like an ominous shadow over the future of humanity. Only cooperation holds back these weapons of mass destruction.

Genes may be behind these worldwide problems, and human culture may also be to blame, but both offer hope. According to Dawkins, we are genetically predisposed to survive by addressing the barriers we face in our environment. Such survival mechanisms include our ability to learn from our past and simulate our possible future as a means to prepare for a better tomorrow.

The *cultural soup*, as Dawkins called it, changes rapidly. Culture, for now at least, is outpacing genetics in evolving human behavior, and this could be a good thing, because we may not have much time. Humankind is capable of recognizing an imbalance with its environment, capable of learning from its history, and capable of planning change to support its future.

The question is this: Which future will best serve humankind? Is it a future driven by the masters of selfishness, the Few (individualists pursuing totalitarianism through corporate or communist oligarchy, or by dictatorship) or a future driven by the many (mutualism forming healthy democracy)?

The oligarchs of the world are rapidly moving society toward totalitarianism. Totalitarianism is a form of war culture. Totalitarians are at war with all things they deem a threat. In war culture, being driven by hierarchy is a necessity; the many must act as one body, largely without question. This strategy of strict hierarchy with the use of "us-against-them" memes has proven to be helpful, not only in war but also in business, politics, evangelizing, and advocacy, for example. It is not a strategy to be totally disregarded. The cultures that deploy it most effectively tend to subjugate those that do not. In many ways, it is what has brought humanity to world domination and now offers humanity the prizes of vast materialism and technological splendor, at least for some of us.

The problem is this: to be good at war, a group must be good at dehumanizing others. This dehumanization process, in social psychology terms, is what makes war largely possible. If a zero-sum culture (war culture) dominates a society, the dehumanization of others will follow, and the members of that society will tend to seek out warlike activity against each other whenever there is diversity. War culture is a culture of division—us against them, the in-group versus the out-group. It is a zero-sum game, and ultimately our divisions will cause our democracy to fall.

Conversely, to be good at waging peace, a group must be good at humanizing others, even those perceived as enemies. Jesus asked his followers to "love thine enemy." Peace culture is the culture of unity. Unity culture is a win-win proposition. Healthy democracy brings balance between these diametrically opposed cultures because it not only champions individual rights (allowing the dominant individuals opportunity to excel through warlike (competitive) culture, but is also built on the premise that all humans are created equal (affording the majority, less-dominant, citizens protections against oppression). The commitment to equality and individual rights offers society balance, and healthy democracy offers both.

The problem with the Few driving the colony is that their collective consciousness is pathologically motivated by the attributes of the selfish gene as identified by Dawkins (1989), or Townsend's (2003) aggressive, ruthless, greedy, presocial minds. Ultimately, these tendencies will encourage the Few to serve the Few at the expense of the many. This is what they have always done, this is what they have evolved to do better than the many, and this is why they are the Few. Being led by utter selfishness has been the downfall of entire civilizations.

Jared Diamond in his 2005 book *Collapse: How Societies Choose to Fail or Succeed* uses the Prisoner's Dilemma experiments to describe a strategy that past societies have used to choose collapse. Essentially, the Few (my term) and their alliances will tend to choose defection instead of collaboration. In numerous examples, Diamond described how populations and their leaders identified the problem threatening their civilization as greed and selfishness and still chose to fail. For example, societies have chosen to deplete fish populations or forests, or overuse soil through agriculture in order to personally gain— knowingly, to the detriment of everyone else, even the entire civilization.

On the other hand, if the colony (Townsend's term) is truly driven by mutualism, it will be forced to serve the many through social mind attributes. The assumption here is that, given the right leadership and environment, it is more likely that the many, through preprogrammed and programmed values based on mutualism, will be motivated to guide overall human behavior toward the common good. They will then build a society of the many, by the many, and for the many— a society based more on reciprocal altruism—that is, a healthy democracy.

The many are largely expendable to the Few; at least they are much more expendable to the Few than to the many themselves. Indulge me in this fantasy to illustrate the point: how many people on Earth does it take to maximize the life of the Few? As technology evolves, the need for workers diminishes. The more people there are, the more they demand resources of the world and therefore fewer resources are available to the Few. Is the answer zero population growth? How about a twenty-five or even a fifty percent reduction of the population? Remember that the selfish gene, the animal and primordial minds, are utterly ruthless. Unless other humans are part of a close genetic relationship, as far as the base impulse of the selfish gene is concerned, they are merely part of the environment. They either get in the way, or they exist to be exploited. The many are difficult to manage. Historically (other than like-kind rivals of the Few), the many are the greatest threat to human organizations that are driven by the Few. The many foster revolutions, unions, inclusive populism, and, of course, democracy.

By withholding medicines, instituting austerity, encouraging abortion, fostering military policy in Africa that leads to starvation and energy policy in the United States that exacerbates climate change, the Few could shrink the gene pool. Fomenting civil disorder and race and religious wars as well as creating an industrial prison/slave/war complex-based society would help reduce population as well. It's a very ugly way to achieve a more manageable world or population control, but for the Few, through the presocial mind, the base attributes of the selfish gene would have no conscience with respect to these matters.

Should the remaining human beings be left to their own devices? Why should this potential threat be left to fester and grow? The presocial mind, the selfish gene, is greedy; it is interested in the resources of others. It is also fearful. The remaining population must be put to use, or put to death. Those who serve the all-powerful Few will be allowed to procreate. Those who fail to do so will be destroyed. This strategy includes the above methods of purging the Earth of humanity, and also genetic manipulation. Genetic manipulation could weed out rebellious genes. Why not take this step, if it is at the disposal of the all-powerful Few? Remember that the presocial minds don't have a conscience. The selfish gene orientation is ruthless. Under utter dominance of the Few, the concept of *designer babies* takes on an all-new meaning.

These possibilities are not baseless. Totalitarians—both fascist and communists—have already pursued these ends. Creating a genetic "new man" was a goal of Adolf Hitler. Edvins Snore's (2008) documentary *The Soviet Story* reminds us that Karl Marx and Vladimir Lenin advocated class genocide in order to create the new man culturally. In both cases, the new man would fulfill the goals established by the Few. Snore quotes Marx: "The classes and the races too weak to master the new conditions of life must give way . . . They must perish in the revolutionary Holocaust." Snore documented how, under Stalin, the Soviet Union ruthlessly followed this horrific doctrine by systematically starving to death seven million Ukrainians.

On the other hand, the many truly in control of the many are forced to respect the self-determination of one another. In the past, the problem has been that attempts that promote the collective agenda such as government ideologies (e.g., communism, socialism, and democracy) in the end tend to be driven by the Few. For the world to achieve a process where the many truly determine the common good would be more than revolutionary—it would have to be evolutionary. Cultural evolution is what is needed.

Remember, according to Sapolsky (2005), environment largely triggers the genetic and nervous system activity responsible for human behavior. It appears that, from the wilderness of prehistoric times to the glass and concrete inner cities of urban America, our environments have brought out, dangerously, the baser characteristics innate in our human biology responsible for behavior. Although the approach of conquering others in order to form empires, nations, or even markets and maintaining control through guile and coercion has brought Americans, Europeans, and indeed much of the world many beneficial innovations and luxuries, this behavior could be rapidly bringing us toward our own demise.

Perhaps "survival of the fittest" and the "meek shall inherit the Earth" are two conceptual beacons that have merged into an overarching call to humanity—a mundane strategy for human survival? Surviving for the many could mean being meek enough to authentically collaborate with diversity on a vast scale never before achieved—a new macroculture that inspires the more reciprocal, altruistic side of human biology.

Ironically, war culture has not only brought the clash of diversity to new heights, it has brought us new hope. War culture has expanded its reach to all corners of the Earth, but it has brought Christ with it, in a sense. It has connected the peoples of the world, and in so doing has opened channels to the potential for empathy and community never before achieved on Earth.

Our charge as stewards of the Earth is to manage not only complexity but also variety (diversity). The easiest way to do this is through authoritarian rule. But the effectiveness of such an approach is limited. Authoritarian process manages diversity by suppressing expression. But diversity is not always eliminated by suppression; it often remains festering in search of expression that could erupt into violent revolution. Authoritarians of the Super Cheats class understand this, and that, in part, can lead them to committing genocide—"if the threat does not exist, it cannot revolt."

The impulse to compete with diversity may be rooted in our genetics. We are designed to compete in order to replicate our memes and genes. But evolution also requires variety (diversity). Without diversity of genes and memes, we limit our ability to adapt to our ever-changing environment, and we are threatened with the dead end of our own evolution. That is why we are also designed to cooperate. We must continue to evolve, mimetically (culturally) as a matter our survival. Moreover, I believe it is possible to guide our cultural evolution to enhance the prospects of our biological evolution. This belief is a view disparaged by mainstream proponents of evolutionary psychology, however, I'm not alone in this assessment. According to Richerson and Boyd (2005, 192-193)

> Natural selection, mutation, and drift shape gene frequencies, while natural selection, guided variation, and variety of transmission biases mold the distribution of cultural variants. However, these two processes are not independent. Each partner of the coevolutionary dance influences the evolutionary dynamics of the other.

In order to be effective stewards of the Earth and the future of humanity, the many must manage the guided variation and variety of transmission biases instead of the Few (i.e., class of Super Cheats). We have organized our societies largely based on war culture driven by the Few. We must now organize society based on healthy democracy—a more empathetic, reciprocal–altruistic social order.

If the human environment (prehistoric, feudalistic, imperialistic, fascist, materialistic) has encouraged the selfish, deceitful, coercive, and murderous side of humanity, what environment can encourage a more loving, just, altruistic side to humanity—one more conducive to healthy democracy? Surely, environments exist that encourage such behavior outside of those comprising individuals with close genetic ties. Could such an environment potentially affect other environments to adopt similar values or at least practices? The ultimate prize would be if this more reciprocal–altruistic environment could spread its practices and values to government and consequently the corporate sector, altering the underpinning culture of society. I submit that such environments exist and that we are pursuing the development of such environments, not only one person at a time but also one organization at a time. If we could identify and encourage such microculture development, perhaps we could ultimately encourage the organization of healthier democracy in our communities, nation, and perhaps one day even the world based on that model.

The question is this: what environment could encourage a more reciprocal–altruistic side to human nature and serve as the soil for the cultivation of healthy democracy worldwide? This environment would, presumably, have to be fundamentally altruistically oriented, possessing a worldwide scope and major economic significance. It would likely involve all races, religions, and classes, and it would transcend national boundaries. Focused on the concerns of the many, it would operate closely with the many to provide fertile ground for widespread participation in solving the problems of the many.

Ironically, such an environment may be right under our noses. It has emerged in response to the failure of governments to propagate a more altruistic society and as a counterforce to the growing dominance of industry the world over. The environment that is being alluded to is the nonprofit or not-for-profit sector.

The not-for-profit sector is a facet of world society comprising organizations structured in many ways. But what these organizations have in common are missions that strive to altruistically serve. Consequently, not-for-profit organizations draw participation in the form of donations and volunteerism—and grassroots workers who often, themselves, benefit from the missions of these organizations. This encourages the organizations to be of the people, by the people, and for the people they serve. The not-for-profit sector offers environments motivated by empathy and therefore fertile ground for equity—the root of healthy democracy.

CHAPTER 13

The Reciprocal–Altruistic Sector of Society: Fertile Soil for Healthy Democracy?

MAXWELL S. KENNERLY posted the following on his blog in 2010:

> Under eBay v. Newmark, the law is as [Senator] Franken said: "it is literally malfeasance for a [for-profit] corporation not to do everything it legally can do to maximize its profits.". . . The impact of this duty-to-maximize-profits stretches far beyond mere investments. Under Citizens United [ruling], corporations now have the First Amendment right to influence our fragile democracy however they want, since they're "people" just like you and me, albeit profit-maximizing zombies who care not for truth, justice, or the American way.

For-profit corporations and their cultural values increasingly serve as the underpinning of our environment, and this has an effect on our reality. These corporations largely control society's information, economics, and leaders, as well as our state and federal governments. Corporate culture is becoming the American culture, the culture of maximizing personal profit at all costs.

Creating healthy democracy requires overturning the laws and traditions that promote short-term profit above all else. This is an immense and overwhelming undertaking that must be pursued. If we are to heal humanity psychologically, culturally, and spiritually, we need an environment that encourages reciprocity as opposed to selfishness. Reciprocity is what holds together healthy democracy. The nonprofit or not-for-profit sector offers hope for being such a countervailing force against selfishness in the world, because its nature is to give.

Unlike our federal government and increasingly, our state and local governments, our grassroots not-for-profits remain overwhelmingly in the hands of everyday people. This means that a major portion of society's organizational capacity is still in our control, and we can build on this. For those of us engaged in the not-for-profit sector, one of the things we can do is to begin to create healthy democracy in the organizations where we work or volunteer. As difficult as this work to achieve greater democracy can be in our not-for-profit organizations, it is, for many of us, a tangible means of expanding democracy and contributing toward a social environment that counters corporate greed. If healthy democracy in our nonprofit sector was widely spread, this could even help influence greater reciprocity in for-profit corporations (I will explore how this might work in later chapters.).

For most of us, it is not practical to try to bring attention to, let's say, General Electric's maximization of profits at the expense of the United States Treasury (i.e., paying zero federal taxes), or to compete with their lobbyists on issues revolving around corporate taxation (although these approaches are also absolutely necessary). It is more practical for some of us to help expand democracy one procedure or policy or program at a time in our own organizations. Ideally, many of us will eventually transform our entire organization into an effective, efficient democracy. By pursuing healthy democracy one organization at a time, we are able to gain ground toward a healthy democracy on a practical basis.

The Reciprocal–Altruistic Sector of Society: Fertile Soil for Healthy Democracy?

Organizations are made up of subsystems (e.g., accounting, marketing, programs, fundraising). If we examine the state of the subsystems of an organization, we see the state of that organization. If we change the subsystems of an organization, we change the organization. Likewise, society is made up of numerous organizations of all kinds (not-for-profit, for-profit, government), and in a sense, they are the subsystems of our society. The collective state of those organizations reveals the state of the given society. If we change the organizations of society, we change society. We can engage in this process by changing the organizations that are under our control within the not-for-profit sector, as this sector is more accessible to this change than the for-profit sector. The current political system in the United States is extremely resistant to healthy democracy as a consequence of legalized political bribery and the two-party, winner-take-all system and corporate influence.

The not-for-profit sector, if highly democratized, could serve as a powerful countervailing force against the dehumanization imposed by corporate culture. Although it can be argued that not every not-for-profit organization can logically be democratized, it is the contention set forth in this book that the (healthy) democratization of the sector could potentially become the rule if so chosen by its participants and could serve as a central part of a movement that causes the United States to evolve toward becoming a healthier democracy. For example, not-for-profit organization at the grassroots level could anchor the social justice movements emerging in America in the values and norms of healthy democracy, thereby orienting and socializing its participants in healthy democracy.

If there is a sector of society that is anywhere close to Christ like in its purpose and, at the same time, is pluralistic (inclusive of all religions and humanistic creeds), it would have to be the not-for-profit sector. With the greatest focus on religious work, education, human service, public benefit, and health, the sector espouses values that are highly altruistic. The not-for-profit sector seeks to educate the poor, heal the sick, feed the hungry, clothe the naked, support the imprisoned, advocate for peace, embrace the stranger, and save the souls of humanity.

If we could develop our most powerful for-profit organizations, from media to multinational corporations and banks, to be structured in a manner that adopts more of the values of the not-for-profit sector as a precondition to operations—providing them with a dual bottom line of altruistic service and profit, we would be structuring our environment to, in large part, perpetuate social responsibility and encourage empathy—the gateway to agape love. We see this emerging possibility with the advent of the B Corporation that is structured to pursue both profit and altruism. Furthermore, if the requirements for allowing these major corporations to operate included an increasing level of democratization that corresponds to the influence the industry has on the commons, we could radically change the direction of society. Perhaps whenever a major corporation, by its nature, has wide ranging influence on our democracy, it would be required to be a not-for-profit as well. We can see such organizations emerging in society throughout the world. Many of today's businesses are not-for-profits, such as hospitals, insurance companies, banks, and grocery stores. Some countries (e.g., Germany) require workers to sit on the advisory board of directors of certain industries and elect the board of directors of the companies where they work. They also require these industries to answer to local democratic bodies before making certain major business decisions. Democratically structured cooperatives are emerging around the world. These businesses offer efficiency, economic development, and worker empowerment. But in order to move forward with a more empathetic and democratic economy, we must also establish strong organizations that promote social change that are themselves rooted in the lives and explicit requirements of the everyday man, woman, and child that they serve through democratic process. Healthy democratic not-for-profit organizations that exist today can help achieve a healthy democracy for our nation.

Perhaps at one point in our history, American for-profit corporations were, at least superficially, legally obliged to give back to society.

The Reciprocal–Altruistic Sector of Society: Fertile Soil for Healthy Democracy?

Today the idea of for-profit corporate responsibility is legalistically diminished. Since our government is now under the control of its corporate overseers, we have much work to do within the not-for-profit sector to balance corporate influence. However, private charitable not-for-profit organizations (and nonincorporated groups) with values and works rooted in healthy democratic norms offer hope. This hope is elevated in concert with individuals living socially responsible lives and who passively resist corporate domination and pursue change geared toward a healthy democratic reality. Together these two fronts of our cultural evolution, if converged, would provide the foundation for a successful political revolution that offers control of the pillars of power to the everyday citizen.

Defining the Sector

What exactly constitutes a not-for-profit organization is subject to contention, as is the true value of the not-for-profit organization to society. In 1999, the Johns Hopkins Center for Civil Society Studies published *Global Civil Society: Dimensions of the Nonprofit Sector.* This publication offered some parameters, or five common characteristics, that help define the sector. (Salamon et al. 1999, 3-4).

1. Organizations—they have an institutional presence and structure.
2. Private—they are institutionally separate from the state.
3. Not profit distributing—they do not return profits to their managers or to a set of owners.
4. Self-governing—they are fundamentally in control of their own affairs.
5. Voluntary—membership in them is not legally required and they attract some level of voluntary contribution of time or money.

The study divided the sector into twelve fields of function: culture/recreation, education and research, health, social services, environment, development, civic and advocacy, philanthropy, international, religious congregations, business/professional/unions, and other. The study focused on twenty-two countries in Europe, Latin America, and the Middle East as well as the United States. It found that the not-for-profit sector is a major economic force that, even with the exclusion of religious congregations, represents 4.6% of these countries' gross national products. Even without volunteers, the sector in each country studied employs more people than the largest private business in each of their respective countries. The largest overall areas of employment in the not-for-profit sector are education (30%), health (20%), and social service (18%).

Furthermore, the John Hopkins study revealed that most of the revenue of the not-for-profit sector overall comes from fees and charges (49%), with the second largest share of revenue (40%) coming from the public sector, and the smallest share (11%) coming from philanthropy. In fact, none of the countries in the study had revenues dominated by philanthropy.

Not-for-profit organizations are known by many names, among them third-sector organizations, nongovernmental organizations (NGOs), and volunteer organizations. The not-for-profit sector is often referred to as the tax-exempt sector, civil society sector, commons, charitable sector, nonproprietary sector, volunteer sector, or nonprofit sector. Because not-for-profit organizations can be defined legalistically as tax-exempt organizations, they are usually called nonprofits in the United States (Hall 2005).

Sjostrand (1999) discussed not-for-profit organizations at great length. He noted that they can be said to exist without any legal structure. They can be viewed as empirical entities, that is, as a set of planned human interactions regardless of legal structure. They can also be described as theoretical constructs. Even the reasons for the existence of the sector altogether are contentious. For example, the not-for-profit sector could have emerged due to the failures of government, or of the marketplace, or even the family. He discussed the way some theorists (e.g., Hodgson 1987; Etzioni 1988; Anheier 1990; Sjostrand 1995) have

The Reciprocal–Altruistic Sector of Society: Fertile Soil for Healthy Democracy?

veered away from these essentially functional views in explaining the reason for the emergence of the not-for-profit sector. These alternative views include "a focus on the individual stressing complexity . . . those which only promote self-interest (and lead to material, status-oriented, or personal utilities), but also those which exclusively contribute to the utilities of others (i.e., pure altruism)" (Sjostrand 1999, 9).

Sjostrand also noted that others have suggested that the sector might exist not so much because of a failure, but because of human relations and asymmetries (e.g., power relationships) or symmetry (e.g., networking).

In essence, these varying views about the reason for the not-for-profit sector's existence represent diverse beliefs and assumptions about the world. The constructs that derive from these views also help form the basis of the relationships that establish individual organizations throughout the sector. That is, organizations are made up of human relationships, and human relationships in not-for-profits are based in large part on beliefs and assumptions about the world. Sjostrand (1999, 16) explored relationships in the context of human organization, saying that

> Ideal-based rationality copes with uncertainty by uniting individuals who are not acquainted with each other, on the basis of explicit, common values. These shared values and ideals establish a sense of trust which bridges human, geographical, and temporal gaps/distances. Organizing on the basis of common ideals primarily gives individuals a feeling of participation in (some) human ideals and this provides a social and cultural identity. Ideals unite unrelated individuals and provide a shared context.

This description of ideal-based rationality illustrates how relationships that involve common interests at the organizational level serve as the basis for the organization. These relationships may be established under the auspices of a not-for-profit organization for many reasons, including the failure of government or the need for a counterbalance to oligarchic for-profit corporate structures. Nonetheless, underlying these functional purposes are the values of the individuals who pursue the goals of the organization. Common values spawn relationships that, in turn, serve as the fabric of the not-for-profit organization and relate to the pursuit of its mission.

Pertinent Not-for-profit Sector Directions

Strategic alliances are taking on more importance in today's not-for-profit sector. By the end of the Twentieth Century strategic alliances had become a valued methodology for success in the not-for-profit sector. Yankey and Willen (2005, 257) described strategic alliances, also known as collaboration and strategic restructuring, as "capacity-building mechanisms that enable partnering entities to achieve results exceeding those that might be attained on the basis of each participant's individual resources and efforts."

Strategic alliances exist along a continuum of formalization, from collaboration of separate entities to integration of two or more organizations into one. Yankey and Willen (2005, 258-259) used the Partnership Matrix created by David La Piana (1999) to illustrate this continuum. In the Partnership Matrix, collaboration is shown indicating the greatest level of autonomy. Examples of collaborations include "information sharing, mutual support, and development of executives, some joint purchasing, program coordination, and joint planning." Characteristics of collaboration are shown to include "no permanent organizational commitment" and "decision-making power remains with the individual organizations."

Yankee and Willen also described the next items along the continuum of the Partnership Matrix. Strategic alliance includes administrative consolidation (e.g., contracting for services, sharing services) and joint programming (e.g., single focus or program, multiple focus or program, integrated system). Strategic alliance, according to the Partnership Matrix, "(a) involves a commitment to continue for the foreseeable future, (b) decision-making power is shared or transferred, and (c) is agreement-driven." Then comes the highest level of strategic alliance formalization, corporate integration (e.g., merger, joint venture corporations, and parent/subsidiary). According to the Partnership Matrix, "Corporate integration involves changes to corporate control and/or structure, including creation and/or dissolution of one or more organizations" (2005, 259).

Organizational cooperation in the not-for-profit sector includes government contracts. Over the last thirty or so years, there has been an increase in the government contracting with not-for-profit sector organizations for a variety of reasons, including the government seeking less expensive ways to address social issues and not-for-profits looking for more efficient ways to raise funding (Smith 2005).

One example of a not-for-profit/government contract relationship is the charter school. Charter schools are semiautonomous public schools, founded by educators, parents, community groups, or private organizations that operate under a written contract with a state district or other entity. This contract, or charter, details how the school will be organized and managed, what students will be taught and expected to achieve, and how success will be measured. Many charter schools enjoy freedom from rules and regulations affecting other public schools, as long as they continue to meet the terms of their charters. Charter schools can be closed for failing to satisfy these terms (Education Commission of the States 2005, 1).

Smith (2005, 374) compared the relationship of not-for-profits and government to regimes:

> Regimes tend to have accepted means of resolving disputes and addressing particular problems . . . The regime concept is helpful in illuminating the regularized patterns of interaction between government and nonprofit agencies, even when these nonprofit organizations are opposed or resistant to government regulations and mandates. Participants are mutually dependent and marked by continuity . . . if participants depart from the regime norms, they are penalized, either by the dominant party

[in this case government] or third parties. Regimes are usually sustained and dominated by a powerful party.

Smith noted how generally like-minded individuals committed to a common issue(s) create not-for-profits, particularly small not-for-profit organizations. The functions are supported by in-kind and small cash donations. They are also typically undercapitalized and can be significantly affected by disruptions in cash flow. Consequently, managers of not-for-profits with government contracts tend toward being beholden to the government administrator's goals, which can lead not-for-profits away from their missions. Under these circumstances, many not-for-profit organization managers find themselves trapped because private funding is inadequate.

Because of the intense competition for government contracts among not-for-profit organizations, management is under greater pressure to be mistake free, or the contract may be lost to a competitor. To address these circumstances, Smith suggested that not-for-profit organizations recruit board members with knowledge of government contracts as well as community members who can provide feedback regarding the organization's performance. Smith also described a need to expand the agency's constituency. Many not-for-profit organizations boast boards of directors that do not represent the larger community and so miss an opportunity for greater assistance.

Smith recommended that a not-for-profit enlarge its constituency by joining community organizations, altering its rules of membership, or creating advisory councils. He encouraged not-for-profits to seek politicians and their friends to serve on their boards, to engage in public relations activities geared toward politicians, and to join associations that influence government. He also asserted that advocacy is emerging as a trend in the not-for-profit sector. Further, due in no small part to contracting with government, more not-for-profit organizations are tied to the political process. As a consequence, these organizations are more motivated to engage in political advocacy. Smith (2005, 383) also asserted that enlarging constituencies might also pose problems:

Enlarging the agency's constituency through these new initiatives or governance structures is not without risks. New members or supporters may try to change the agency's mission and lead it in new directions. An agency may trade dependency on state contract administrators for dependency on a powerful donor or group of donors.

Growth of the Not-for-profit Sector and Its Role in Society

Anecdotally, the not-for-profit sector's flexibility and arguably less costly participatory approach enable it to do more with less than can government. Therefore, theoretically speaking, the not-for-profit sector can serve as a counterforce to government failure to meet the requirements of its citizenry beyond the privileged classes (Salamon 1999). But this is far from a proven fact. According to Cross (1997, 4), the not-for-profit sector may be subject at times to the political agendas of both liberal and conservative elements while being limited in its ability to politically advocate on behalf of their program beneficiaries. He described how this could be occurring:

> Donors with a liberal agenda, or who want to appear liberal, therefore often justify the funneling of resources through NGOs on the assumption that this will develop political institutions in civil society. On the other hand, the notion that NGOs increasingly take over the welfare role of the state—providing support for the poor and development for the country—this process complements the growing emphasis on privatization and decentralization of state functions. Civil society appears capable of taking care of its own needs, according to this argument, providing added impetus to those who argue that the role of the state should be reduced to a minimum . . . Very often, state regulation implies that local

NGOs and, even more so, international NGOs often have to remain apolitical in order to retain their status. The problem emerges when one considers the possible variations in the term political activism. Is it just when you support a candidate for public office, or does it extend to situations such as lobbying for new laws or helping to organize the poor better represent their own interests?

According to Cross, the trend in the sector has been one of co-option and counter co-option. First, conservative charity programs such as religious groups were co-opted by left-wing entities in order to develop resistance to oppression from below, and then, a right-wing hijacking occurred of the left-wing structure by substituting neoliberal strategies such as antiwelfarism and antistatism. Cross (1997, 5-6) also challenged the notion of not-for-profit organizations always being aligned with the masses:

> The ideal that NGOs represent civil society while states represent elites is predicated on the argument that NGOs are potentially more participatory than the state and market structures, and therefore potentially more accountable to the needs of [lower socioeconomic classes] in society. This provides them with greater legitimacy in representing the needs of society, or at least of the masses . . . Not only are NGOs better than the state from this perspective, but by extension, local NGOs are better than international NGOs . . . Both claims may have some merit, but at the same time they should not necessarily be taken at face value . . . Foley (1996), for example, points out that the role of outside donor organizations in El Salvador is heavily political in focus . . . Far from being participatory, these groups were typically allied with the business elite in the country, which the U.S. was eager to foster.

The Reciprocal–Altruistic Sector of Society: Fertile Soil for Healthy Democracy?

Cross eventually argued that the perception that not-for-profit organizations are more efficient, innovative, and flexible because of their independence from government bureaucracy may not be entirely true. To the extent that these claims are true, they may be attributed to other reasons. Flexibility in not-for-profit organizations, according to Cross, may actually mean they are easier for elite groups to manipulate as compared to local governments. Cross asserted that, furthermore, the larger, more professionalized not-for-profit organizations (that is, large-budget not-for-profits organized more like corporate businesses) are often more dependent on outside funding and are less innovative and flexible than those that are not.

Cross (1997, 9) concluded that there is lack of agreement in the literature regarding the benefits of not-for-profit organizations. Not-for-profits theoretically can provide a host of benefits to society, "But in practice, the larger NGOs grow, the less accountable they are to their beneficiaries and the more accountable they are to the donors who allow them to grow."

Smith (2005) encouraged expanding not-for-profit organization constituencies in order to support partnerships with government agencies and other funding sources, yet Cross stressed the danger of co-option that can result from such partnerships. While recognizing the possibility of cross-sector as well as other partnerships affecting the focus of not-for-profit organizations as Cross suggested, Smith's underlying point is that the quality of the partnership, not the concept of cross-sector partnership itself, should be the issue.

Dependence theory supports Smith's recommendations with respect to approaching relationships that organizations such as not-for-profits have with aspects of their environment, including other not-for-profits, corporate funders, and government contracts. According to the theory, organizations are controlled by their environments, but can influence counterdependence in order to establish more self-determination (Pfeffer and Salanck 1978). This view encourages organizations to identify their critical resources and manage their resource dependencies. With increased not-for-profit advocacy, the advent of crowd-sourcing, social media, and increasing strategic alliances, not-for-profit organizations today have more options than ever to leverage resources that protect their independence. It is incumbent on these organizations to vigorously pursue these methods for establishing resources. The potential for not-for-profit organizations to remain independent rests in their ability to manage their dependencies. Those that succeed in this effort are more apt to remain true to their missions and constituencies and realize the participatory potential of the sector.

In the view of population ecology or organizational ecology, the environment, in a sense, selects successful organizations based on its needs. According to population ecology, the evolutionary processes of selection, variation, and retention explain the relationship between organizations and their environments (Hannan and Freeman 1989). The public is a major part of the environment of the organizations within a given society, and we, the people, largely choose which ones we want to succeed. By donating to not-for-profits whose missions we support as well as advocating for their funding and for them to be more democracy oriented, we can shape and promote them. But choosing organizations also involves more than buying from them or donating to them or even advocating for their change from the outside; it also involves shaping those organizations from within the organizations as members, volunteers, and staff. Grassroots organizations are *our* organizations. They are still under our control. To maximize their focus on the needs of the people they serve involves strategic thinking and action.

The focus a not-for-profit organization takes is based on many variables, including the external environment (service recipients, regulators, funders), the values and relationships of the members, organizational mission and vision, finance, structure, and staff. In order to develop healthy democracy in our not-for-profit organizations and consequently the sector, we must, as insiders of these organizations, develop ethical practices, performance management, funding strategies, and organizational cultures that support healthy democracy. The most important characteristic in achieving this end is leadership.

Leadership will determine the response to efforts to co-opt each not-for-profit organization—the organization's financial strategy, strategic alliances, performance management, organizational culture and ultimately the sector. The questions then are: What organizational characteristics are more apt to encourage a more reciprocal–altruistic not-for-profit organizational culture? What characteristics are associated with not-for-profit organizations that successfully engage in mutually beneficial alliances that help solve the problems of their program beneficiaries and elevate the participatory nature of the not-for-profit sector? What are the pertinent organizational characteristics for healthy democracy in our not-for-profit organizations, and by extension, our communities and nation?

CHAPTER **14**

Healthy Democracy as Organizational Culture

AFTER REVIEWING HUNDREDS of pertinent research papers and works by subject experts (see the bibliography at the end of this book for more detail), I ascertained numerous organizational characteristics that could serve as part of the fabric of healthy democracy in not-for-profit organizations as well as our government institutions. These characteristics include leaders with a deep connection to the organization's mission and the people the mission serves. The leadership style for healthy democracy would likely exhibit the desire to serve the people first and lead the people second. These leaders would have a strong propensity to build community through the use of win–win solutions, but also capacity for distributive negotiations, when required. The ethics of these leaders would rest on respect for diversity of values among their followers in balance with the commitment to the core value of mutuality among the people served. Moreover, this ethical framework would pursue the maintenance of the will and dignity of those that the leaders profess to serve through strong facilitative skills. We call these leaders *servant leaders* (see Greenleaf, 1970).

A healthy democracy would presumably be rooted in an organizational ethic that beckons to agape love. It would display transparency and exhibit a strong service ethic. Healthy democracy would educate and socialize its members to strengthen interrelationships, cooperation, and value for others. It would even help members of the democracy to transcend their own worldviews (without fearing loss of identity) in order to expand moral awareness and scope of justice.

A healthy democracy would presumably be like a quality culture.[6] It would encourage the pursuit of quality worlds[7] of its workers and those that the democracy serves, and it would be structured to be effective and efficient and continuously improving in its pursuit of mission in service to the people. In support of the quality worlds of the people, healthy democracy would likely exhibit a value for procedural justice for staff and program beneficiaries as well as advocacy on behalf of those it represents with respect to issues pertaining to the organization's mission. Nonetheless, healthy democracy would shy away from "us-against-them" views of external as well as internal relationships.

Healthy democracy would presumably operate as if change is a part of life and would be organized to manage change proactively. Change would likely be seen as evolution, and continuous improvement would be among its goals. Small groups and organizations would help facilitate this evolution and innovation, and social entrepreneurship[8] would likely be a featured means to answering the problems posed by change and the service recipient's requirements.

Finally, healthy democracy would presumably use program beneficiary involvement throughout its affairs. It would involve constituencies in creating policy and program development in order for them

---

6 A culture that is results and customer focused, rooted in employee involvement, partnership development, continual improvement, management by fact, leadership-established unity of purpose and a long-range view of the future.

7 According to Glasser (1995) quality is built into the genetic structure of the human brain and is subsumed by five basic needs: survival, love/belonging, power/recognition, freedom, and fun. One's *quality world* is the satisfaction achieved with the given experiences in life.

8 According to Light (2006), social entrepreneurial characteristics are based on the characteristics of entrepreneurs, but are played out in the context of addressing social problems. Social entrepreneurs have the attributes of business entrepreneurs but are focused on achieving community betterment, and caring for and helping people as opposed to establishing successful profit-making ventures.

to pursue mutually desired outcomes and build communities that respect diverse interests within the framework of the given mission of the organization.

After my involvement as a paid consultant in a number of research projects that examined not-for-profit organizations with respect to issues of management and diversity, as well as decades of experience working as a social entrepreneur and administrator of not-for-profit organizations, I designed and implemented a formal research project that focused on involvement of not-for-profit beneficiaries in shaping not-for-profit programming. My research sought to identify characteristics associated with not-for-profit organizations that successfully involve their service recipients in shaping the quality of their programs. What began my academic journey to address problems posed by human diversity working together led to exploration of characteristics that could help organizations equitably achieve the actions and programs required of their diverse constituents. I focused on ascertaining a rich, detailed description and framing of the pertinent characteristics.

I identified three small not-for-profits boasting a variety of diversity (class, regional, political, ethnic, racial, gender, gender orientation). The budgets of these organizations ranged from $200,000 to $650,000 annually. In one case (an advocacy organization), funding was derived exclusively through dues, and in another case (a charter school) a combination of government, foundations, and individuals was the source of income. The third not-for-profit that I researched (an art organization with political aspirations) was funded by foundations, sales, and memberships. Two of these case study organizations (the advocacy organization and the charter school) were deemed by their constituents to be highly successful at incorporating their constituents' requirements in the shaping of the programs. Document reviews and participant observation supported the constituents' assertion. Overall, the diversity involved was served equitably. To be clear *equitably* does not necessarily mean *uniformly*, but rather based on an agreed process of service distribution. The third case study organization (the arts organization) had made a valiant effort to do the same, but failed over the course of its history and eventually folded due to a clash between constituencies among other issues.

All three of these organizations were professionalized organizations with college-educated staffs. They maintained close relationships with their constituencies because they were structured to specifically do so. Each had a board of directors with program beneficiary majority quorums that elected officers, of which the chair was required to be representative of the service recipients. These boards of directors selected their successors from families or constituent groups who would put forth volunteers that represented their perspectives. Leadership by women played a predominant role in all three organizations. All three had mission statements and literature that suggested they were services and recipient-focused, and all three pursued broad service recipient participation in establishing their organization's programs, policies, procedures, and affairs.

During the course of the three and a half or so years of my study, never once did I hear the participants of my study describe themselves as democracies, nor did such a description appear in their literatures. Yet whenever I observed the decision-making processes of the successful organizations of my study or whenever they described themselves verbally or in written form, the practices for determining the policies and affairs of their organizations were structured in a way highly consistent with participatory democratic process. These organizational cultures appeared to be producing democracy: a highly effective and efficient form of democracy.

I pursued these case studies using interviews, document reviews, and participant observation. I focused my questioning on many of the presumptive healthy democracy characteristics mentioned above (quality and performance management, community building and collaboration, ethics, leadership style, entrepreneurship, program beneficiary involvement). I compared the salient characteristics of all three of these organizations to determine which were *most* associated with successfully involving their constituents in shaping the programs and activities (and subsequently the policies and affairs) of these organizations.

I then assembled the characteristics most associated with successfully involving the service recipients in shaping the programs of the organizations in my study into the framework of an organizational culture. What I ascertained were the values, the beliefs and assumptions, the norms and cultural artifacts of highly effective, efficient forms of participatory organizations that use a deliberative, democratic process of decision-making to set policy and manage their affairs.

The organizational cultural model derived was effectively and efficiently of, by, and for all the people served by the organization in an equitable way. Furthermore, rooted in the values and norms of this organizational cultural model, one could clearly glean the essence of what Christians call the Golden Rule in the context of the operations. This is not a culture of love per se, but it is a culture that encourages understanding and consideration across the considerable diversity of membership of these organizations. This encouragement lays the foundation for empathy and in so doing encourages a value that is universal among the great religions of the world: love.

The name I have chosen for this organizational cultural model is *Healthy Democracy* (albeit at the microcultural level). I propose that the characteristics associated with the Healthy Democracy model could be used to guide us in developing greater democracy in not-for-profits throughout the sector as well as in our communities and nation.

It must be noted that the successful organizations of my study were far from utopias. Although very successful in their own rights, these were normal-appearing organizations. They faced the same daily struggles within their organizations as other similar not-for-profits. There were tensions with respect to what faction got what resources, and clashes of culture, class, gender identity, race, and region. These organizations struggled with aspects of their external environment for resources and support, as is typical of not-for-profits working in their respective fields. Yet the organizational behavior of these agencies, rooted in the Healthy Democracy model, managed these obstacles while keeping the organizations focused on their missions and the explicit requirements of the beneficiaries of those missions. These organizations also tended to gain greater support from their environment as time passed and even influenced government and other organizations within their community to adopt cultural memes and artifacts based on their organizational cultures.

Two organizational concepts frame the Healthy Democracy model. First, following Weeks and Galunic (2003, 1), not-for-profits that successfully involve program beneficiaries in shaping the quality of their programs, like all organizations, may be "best thought of as cultures, as social distributions of modes of thought and forms of externalization." Furthermore, following Schein (1992), organizations can be framed by three levels of culture: (a) beliefs and assumptions, (b) norms and values, and (c) cultural artifacts.

Therefore, based on my empirical case study findings, the following set of core common beliefs and assumptions, norms and values, and cultural artifacts emerged. They are being presented here as a theory that can describe organizational culture in not-for-profit organizations that successfully involve program beneficiaries in shaping the quality of their programs, of which the precursor was the beneficiaries shaping the organizations policies and affairs. This organizational culture model is offered as a guide to help us in the development of Healthy Democracy in grassroots organizations, our communities, and nation.

If we consider the following organizational culture as we approach structuring our organizations, and as we hire, train, and socialize leaders and staff (even volunteers), we can create in our not-for-profit organizations the kind of environment that we, the people, require of our government. In so doing, we root our works in the needs of the people we serve, and we take ground on behalf of democracy. We focus consciousness on democracy, and since energy follows consciousness, we help create a Healthy Democratic reality.

The organizational culture I will now describe is based on characteristics most associated with the organizations of my study that successfully involved constituents in shaping the quality of their programs. In this organizational culture, constituents also played a dominant role in creating the policies and guiding the general affairs of these organizations.

Healthy Democracy as an Organizational Culture: Beliefs and Assumptions

1. *The mission is believed to be personally relevant to organizational participants.* The leaders and managers of the Healthy Democracy model hold the assumption that having workers with personal experiences with the demographic that the mission serves is important to the success of the organization. It's as if the ideal candidates for staff and board should feel that their participation is more than a job—it's *personal*. This is not to say that absolutely every participant in the organization must be from the constituency served (sometimes this is not reasonable), but a mission-beneficiary demographic would be apparent in key leadership positions in most cases.
2. *The organization's mission is beneficial to society.* Participants in the organizations that achieve Healthy Democracy in their operations, particularly staff and board members, have a deep belief that the work of the organization is important, not just to them personally, but also to society. Often such a belief emerges from experiences that staff and board have that demonstrate to them the need, and ideally the effectiveness, of the work that the organization pursues.
3. *The organization and its leadership exist for the mission beneficiaries, not the mission beneficiaries for the organization and its leadership.* Building a Healthy Democracy in not-for-profit organizations requires leaders, staff, and volunteers who believe that their involvement in the organization is about

Healthy Democracy as Organizational Culture

serving others. The work is more than a job or a hobby to the ideal candidates of such organizations, and, even more than an opportunity to contribute to society, it's believed by them to be a calling.

4. *Program beneficiaries are worthy of self-determination.* Leaders and workers of organizations that are Healthy Democracies believe that those who benefit from the work of their organization are experts, at least in their own pertinent life experiences. Moreover, it is believed that this expertise should be used to lead the organization in the determination of what is best for the lives of these beneficiaries as it relates to the organization's mission and capacity.

5. *All program beneficiaries of the organization are worthy of respect, and organizational members have an obligation to care about their well-being and human dignity.* One assumption of workers in organizations that are Healthy Democracies is that it's not appropriate to look down on, talk down to, or treat the beneficiaries of the mission with anything but the highest respect. Workers authentically connect to and relate to mission beneficiaries as human beings with a right to inalienable dignity, and this is encouraged across the organization.

6. *Justice permeates the organizational operation, and actions counterintuitive to justice such as envy, pride, greed, and deception are clearly seen as incongruent with participation in the organization.* The staff and executive board leaders of the Healthy Democracy model believe deeply in justice for their members, and it is their assumption that negative motivations and selfish behaviors are destructive to the pursuit of the mission and service to beneficiaries. Such behavior is explicitly and implicitly discouraged. The workers are reasonably compensated per their professional community and commensurate with their contributions. However, in most cases finances are not the primary motivator for employee involvement, as they could often do better financially in other endeavors.

7. *Community service is a virtue.* Whereas many in the for-profit sector view wealth and status as a premier asset, staff and leaders of a Healthy Democracy model view community service as a premier asset in society and gain a sense of satisfaction from service to their community.
8. *It is ethically important for not-for-profits to advocate for their positions and program beneficiaries in the context of their mission.* The leaders and staff in the Healthy Democracy model believe in a strong moral obligation to stand up for what their mission represents and the people that their mission exists to serve. It is an assumption that staff has a responsibility to educate pertinent decision makers when necessary in order to achieve the work that they pursue.
9. *Organizations are open systems.* Staff and board of directors of the Healthy Democracy model believe that organizations function best through effectively interacting with the environment—the supersystem. This includes program beneficiaries, similar organizations, pertinent government agencies, for-profit organizations, and the general public.

Healthy Democracy as an Organizational Culture: Norms and Values

1. *Servant leadership, particularly its facilitative aspects, is evident within the organization's staff and program beneficiary board members.* Barbuda and Wheeler (2007, 2) described the characteristics of servant leadership: "having a calling, listening and empathy, healing, awareness, persuasion, conceptualization, foresight, stewardship, growth and building community." A commitment to equality is also associated with servant leadership (Walker 2006). The characteristics exhibited here are service to others, caring, vision, and empowerment. People are what matters most.
2. *Organizational leadership is adept at establishing sufficient trust across diverse interests.* Leaders of the Healthy

Democracy model have strong facilitative skills. They also tend to have connections among the diverse parties involved, and they often serve as boundary-spanning actors in order to articulate positions that encourage trust. According to Kirby (2006) boundary-spanning actors are those people with a high density of connections within a cluster of social structures. Boundary-spanning actors "are better positioned to recognize good ideas because they have more options to choose from and to integrate...and deliver the idea to its new audience" (p. 9).

3. *Organizational leadership is adept at internal and external relationship building in order to identify and solve joint problems.* The leaders in the Healthy Democracy model are community builders. They understand that there is strength in community and pursue it deliberately and intelligently. By focusing on common interests, leaders are able to solve joint problems.

4. *The executive managers have an institutional power management orientation as opposed to a personal power management orientation.* The managers in the Healthy Democracy model work to inspire staff, board, and external commitment to the mission of the organization, as opposed to loyalty to themselves. They demonstrate, through their actions, their belief that the work of the organization is not about them, but about the mission.

5. *There is a high level of fortitude and zealousness regarding the pursuit of the mission exhibited by organizational leadership.* There are many reasons why the organizational leaders of the Healthy Democracy model are zealous in the pursuit of their organizational missions, but none is probably more important than the connections they have with the people that the mission serves.

6. *A strong work ethic exists among core workers, particularly executive management, field experts, and central board*

leadership. Healthy Democracy is a lot of work. The workers of the Healthy Democracy model often put in extra hours at their positions. Furthermore, hard work is the expectation—everyone is expected to pull his or her share of the load.

7. *A non-zero-sum power inclination among board and staff is normative within the organization*. The members of the Healthy Democracy model look first for win–win situations as they approach problems they face during the pursuit of their missions. Using good research and persuasion, managing by fact, and strong facilitative skills support this orientation.

8. *Redemption is afforded members within the organization, but with clear limitations*. These organizations tend to be forgiving, but more like Dawkins' (1989) description of Grudgers than his Suckers. Connection allows them forgiveness and management by fact, and continuous improvement protects them from abuse.

9. *Organizational members identify with program beneficiaries and treat program beneficiaries the way they would expect to be treated in the context of the organization's mission*. Pyles (2003) spoke about broadening our identity in order to make connections with others. The organizations' members had natural connections with the communities they served, but there was diversity (racial, cultural, political, class, regional) as well. The capacity to understand and find ways to relate to diversity was also foundational to empathizing and respecting beneficiaries. Treating beneficiaries with mutual respect and dignity was important to core members.

10. *Use of program beneficiary-focused approaches is normative within the organization*. A constituent-focused approach to solving problems faced by democratic institutions is largely what makes them healthy. The Healthy Democracy organizational model of successful involvement of program beneficiaries in shaping their programs is the centerpiece of their process for understanding and addressing the requirements

of the people their missions exists to serve. This involvement happens through numerous interactions with program beneficiaries, not just at the policy level of the organization.

11. *The organization demonstrates a clear focus on "internal and external cooperation, learning, process management, continuous improvement, employee fulfillment and customer satisfaction,"* as articulated by Boggs (2004). The organizations in my study whose practices were rooted in the Healthy Democracy model emerged organically as quality cultures. They may not even be aware of the term; however, their practices relate directly to performance management, and their assumptions, norms and values, and cultural artifacts make them recognizable as quality cultures. However, unlike the typical "customer" involvement pursued by TQM practices in the corporate world, these organizations' program beneficiaries also shaped policy through democratically structured processes. The Healthy Democracy model is like a quality culture—it is effective, efficient, and service recipient focused, but it also empowers constituents to shape policy.

12. *There is a strong and evident unity of purpose within the organization.* The mission and service recipient-focused culture of the Healthy Democracy model strongly directs the energy of the participants in a unified manner.

13. *The organization has formal and informal processes to establish and maintain a clear group identity.* The Healthy Democracy model uses board members, staff, and a volunteer orientation process to formally initiate participants into the organization's work. Even so, the informal modeling of values and norms may more thoroughly socialize participants in a manner that focuses them toward norms of behavior and beliefs in organizational philosophy. The Healthy Democracy model includes the implicit and explicit socialization of members into the norms and values of the organizational culture.

14. *The organization demonstrates both product and process orientations.* It's not just a matter of the product that results from organizational efforts (although that is very important); the process is also important to members of the organization. Process affects product. Focusing on process as well as product helps them to do the right things the right way.
15. *Functional authority carries much weight within the organization.* Each person involved in the organization has a level of expertise based on the experiences that they bring to the agency. For example, teachers at schools are authorities on curriculum, and the principal is the administrative authority, whereas the families of the students are the experts specific to the student's needs. Although the Healthy Democracy model utilizes collaboration (among equals), those members with the particular expertise for a given project or issue tend to take the lead in guiding those projects based on that expertise.
16. *Use of partnering is normative within the organization.* Working together helps to make democracy healthy. Without the ability to partner with others, the many are at the whim of the Few. In the Healthy Democracy model, organizations partner with not only those the missions serve, they also use cross-functional teams among staff and among staff and board of directors.
17. *Diverse opinion is authentically valued.* Diverse opinion is an explicit value of board and staff in the Healthy Democracy model. There is an understanding that the beneficiaries of their mission represent diversity in many forms. To value all their constituencies, they must value diverse opinion. Leaders associated with the Healthy Democracy model recognize that innovation is often the result of looking at an issue from many perspectives. Instead of fearing such diversity, these leaders embrace it.
18. *The organization uses elements that can be identified as relating to discourse ethics.* Discourse ethics proposes that

through conversation, society or organizations can collectively establish ethical norms (Racine 2003). With respect and sincerity, as well as with a set of communication standards and argumentative and discourse presuppositions, groups can enhance their social capacity.
19. *The organization uses highly effective and varied communication systems to communicate with organizational members and key external entities.* The Healthy Democracy model uses a variety of written, electronic, and in-person communication methods to relay pertinent information in support of the function of the organization.
20. *Progressive levels of participation for program beneficiaries as well as widespread participation of program beneficiaries in the organizational community are normative.* Not every program beneficiary is going to want to serve on the board of directors, but participation at some level is very important. The Healthy Democracy model offers opportunities to participate in a wide variety of forms geared to realistically accommodate the different interests and capabilities of service recipients to participate in the organization in a meaningful manner.
21. *The use of community organizing and strategic alliances is an ongoing strategy for furthering the organization's mission.* The leaders in the Healthy Democracy model understand that other organizations and community members outside of theirs share common interests with them. They also understand that they could often be more effective working together in pursuit of addressing those common interests. By developing awareness of common problems with others in their environment and jointly planning strategies that strengthen the efforts of the respective organizations, the Healthy Democracy model enhances the organization's effectiveness in pursuit of its missions and goals.
22. *Use of technical assistance is a part of the organization's*

process for achieving its goals. Technical assistance from a variety of sources, including leaders of similar organizations, strategic partners, consultants, local experts, and local political leaders is normative in the Healthy Democracy model.

23. *Staff members are afforded latitude for innovation.* Staff members are allowed to be creative and innovative in their approaches to resolving issues while in pursuit of the organization's mission. Innovations that impact only their daily endeavors may be solo projects; however, as the impact of these innovations touch more program beneficiaries, the more democratized the process becomes. Major innovations involve the board of directors and even the entire community of program beneficiaries.

24. *There exists an active social-entrepreneurial orientation among staff members.* Leadership and staff tend to serve as the primary intrepreneurs (i.e., social-entreprenuers working to create internal innovation). These are creative individuals who take calculated risks (in a supportive environment) to develop programs and projects that address the service recipient needs and expressed requirements.

25. *Ongoing program innovations are characteristic of the organization.* These are organizations that use innovation on an ongoing basis in pursuit of their missions. Not all the innovations have successful outcomes, but they are frugally pursued and well planned and implemented. As a result, many innovations are useful, and those that are not have a minimum negative impact.

26. *The organization has a balanced operation regarding a) low risk/high control vs. high risk/low control; b) high vs. low social context; c) polychronic vs. monochronic; and d) person vs. data-driven decision-making.*

According to Curran (2005, 30), the primary themes in not-for-profit organizational culture are (a) the social context, (b) the level

Healthy Democracy as Organizational Culture

of risk, (c) the use of time, and (d) the connection and commitment to purpose. Curran described social context as high or low: "High means that you do have to know a lot of context to understand and interpret information. Low means you do not have to know much history or context to get involved . . . In general, nonprofits tend to be higher context than business corporations."

Curran noted pros and cons associated with the different levels of social context. In high context communication (e.g., a culture of communication by storytelling), stories can amplify meaning and help connect members' commitment to mission. High social context organizations can also pose problems for outsiders trying to understand how the organization works. Conversely, low context communication can compress more data in ways that promote efficiency and fulfill mission on a larger scale. Curran (2005, 31) said that it can also "distract from the humanity of the operation."

The goal suggested by Curran is finding the correct balance of social context for each given organization. This can be achieved through stakeholder participation in establishing both the currant predominant organizational culture and the vision of what the majority wants the organizational culture to be in the future. The Healthy Democracy model is reasonably balanced in terms of social context.

Curran suggested that not-for-profits also need to find the correct balance for each organization regarding the level of risk in which it is willing to engage. Curran represented risk on a continuum with flexibility (high risk) at one end and control (low risk) at the other, both being important to successful operations. Flexibility includes being open to new trends, needs, and ideas, but too much flexibility could cause an organization to follow trends at the expense of the organization's mission. Low-risk/high-control organizational culture tends to be more consistent, but it often stifles innovation and is too slow to respond to changing environments.

Consistent with the examples provided by Curran of strategies that can be used to bring more organizational cultural balance, the Healthy Democracy model uses minimum hierarchy to increase staff and board input. Consistent with Curran's (2005, 33) suggestion, the Healthy Democracy model uses controlled agendas and time at meetings "in a style that [brings] consensus decisions through specific techniques rather than just letting the loudest voices prevail."

Another important organizational cultural consideration in regard to enhancing not-for-profit organizations is use of time. Curran described two ways people use time: (a) monochronically or linearly—one at a time, one after another; and (b) polychronically or with many things happening at once, with periodic selection of which thing to emphasize at any given time frame. According to Curran, managers can manage by time, or by goals. Managing by time (time sheets, culture of compliance over innovation) provides clarity of roles, and budgets can gain more predictability. However, time-focused management can reduce motivation. Goal-focused management is quite the opposite. It may include flextime schedules and an innovative culture that emphasizes the purpose of actions or self-motivation. Nonetheless, goal-focused management can appear to produce a more chaotic workspace. The Healthy Democracy model appears to bring a reasonable balance to both orientations, but with a leaning toward goal-focused orientation.

Healthy Democracy as an Organizational Culture: Cultural Artifacts

1. *The organization has a clear written mission statement.* The mission is the central boundary-spanning tool. It focuses the energy of the participants, clarifies the goals of innovation, and directs and prioritizes resources.
2. *Written program beneficiary-focused organizational philosophy and operation policy exist within the organization.* It is explicit in the literature of these organizations that their work is focused on the requirements of those they exist to serve. There are a variety of written policies and procedures for collecting data from and interacting with service recipients to ascertain their requirements, and this includes strong program

Healthy Democracy as Organizational Culture

beneficiary involvement in governance.

3. *Written policies and procedures that help institutionalize organizational structure that combines elements of collegial consensus and rational bureaucratic organization approaches exist within the organization.* Examples of this include program beneficiary-dominated governance as a matter of written policy and staff involvement in governance structure. The chairperson of the board of directors is required to be a program beneficiary. The organization also has a quorum that requires a majority of the service recipients. The Healthy Democracy model institutionalizes collaboration driven by the constituents of the organization and staff to develop policy as well as shape programming through democratic process.

4. *The organization maintains job descriptions for all organization core workers, including volunteers and board of directors, as well as written expectations for program beneficiary participation opportunities.* Job descriptions clarify who is responsible for what, help to prevent overlapping of activities, and help keep skills matched to tasks.

5. *Training and orientation manuals are widely distributed among core organizational participants.* These organizations have written procedures for bringing in new members of the organization that help to orient them to the organization's tasks, processes, and culture.

6. *The organization has formally organized cross-functional teams that play a central role in decision-making regarding its activities.* Written policy brings together subject experts (e.g., teachers or lead advocates), along with administrators and program beneficiaries to solve problems and engage in planning.

7. *PDCA-like (plan, do, check and act) cycles and participatory evaluation for utilization are part of written procedure within the organization.* Evaluation is used as a part of continuous improvement. Evaluation use in the Healthy Democracy

model is formative as well as summative. Evaluation can take a variety of other forms as well, such as front-end analysis. The beneficiaries of the work of these not-for-profits are a fundamental part of the evaluation of the organization's activities.

8. *The organization uses written "prevention," conflict analysis, and resolution processes.* Provention, according to Burton (1990), is identifying potential future conflicts and addressing them prior to their becoming problems.
9. *Hiring procedures are followed for organizational and job fit.* The organization hiring procedure is not just for the skill set, but also for the way applicant experiences and orientation are likely to add to the synergism of the operation.
10. *The organization's strategic planning documents evidence a capacity for both political decision-making and rational planning methods for addressing the organization's future.* Bryson (1995, 5) defined strategic planning as "a disciplined effort to produce fundamental decisions and actions that shape and guide what an organization is, what it does, and why it does it." Bryson (1995, 11) described two overall approaches to strategic planning: the rational planning model and the political decision-making model. Rational planning "represents a rational deductive approach to decision-making. It begins with goals, policies, programs, and actions are then deduced to achieve those goals." The political decision-making model, on the other hand is inductive: "Beginning with issues, which by definition involve conflict, not consensus, policies and programs emerge that address issues that are politically acceptable."

Healthy Democracy as an Organizational Culture: Conclusion

In the Healthy Democracy model, we can see energy following consciousness and creating a reality of true democracy. Healthy Democracy exists first in the consciousness (beliefs and assumptions, or worldview) of the participants that directs energy into democratic norms of behavior supported and reinforced by written policy and procedure. In turn, the Healthy Democracy memes, values and norms, and cultural artifacts not only help socialize those involved in the organization toward supporting the goals established through Healthy Democracy, they offer the potential to influence those within the organization's environment to adopt memes and values of the Healthy Democracy that can shape the cultural artifacts of outside agencies (including government, as was the case with the successful organizations of my study.)

If we could transfuse more of the characteristics of the above participatory democratic organizational culture (the Healthy Democracy model) into the American system of democracy, we could hope to realize democracy's greater potential. Through cultural evolution, we can pursue transformation of current society from oligarchy to Healthy Democracy. Healthy Democracy is the authentic vehicle for the American dream. By centering our policy decisions on the sustainable version of that dream, as it is defined by *all of us,* we can make America greater than ever.

CHAPTER **15**

Theory of Healthy Democracy in Not-for-Profit Organization

IT IS PROPOSED that not-for-profit organizations that successfully involve program beneficiaries in shaping the quality of their programs exhibit what Kujala and Lillrank (2004) termed quality cultures. Furthermore, like the description of family-centered[9] schools by Jordan et al. (2001), the participation of program beneficiaries is a partnership between equals (program beneficiaries, executive management, and field experts). These organizations fundamentally involve program beneficiary participation in governance and program development for the purpose of achieving program beneficiary satisfaction. That is, the partnership's focal point or focus is on the program beneficiaries' requirements in regard to continually improving the organization's programs within the context of the mission and organizational capacity. Therefore, a descriptively accurate term for describing this organizational culture is *program beneficiary-focused partnership quality culture*. However, because this term is cumbersome, I propose the initialism HMD (*Healthy (microcultural) Democracy*).

Essentially, it is program beneficiary-focused partnership quality culture that establishes Healthy Democracy at the microcultural level

---

9   In this view, families are seen as the primary decision makers for their children, they are supported as key decision makers in all aspects of school services, and their needs beyond the education of the child are also considered.

(system or organizational level). The theory proposes that not-for-profit organizations that successfully involve their program beneficiaries in shaping the quality of their programs through democratic process that includes shaping policy are fundamentally Healthy (microcultural) Democracies (HMDs). Below is offered a graphic that illustrates the theory of Healthy (microcultural) Democracy.

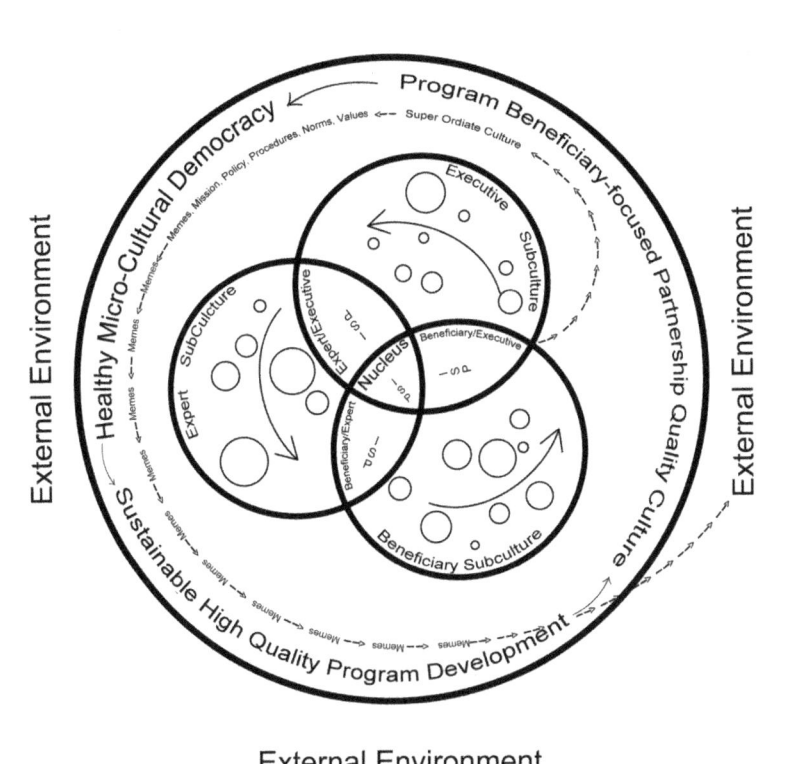

I S P = Informal Subcultural Partnership

FIGURE 1. ISP = Informal subcultural partnership.

Each of the interconnecting spheres represents a subculture within the organization with its own functional authority. There is the expert subculture (e.g., teacher in a school or professional lobbyist in an advocacy organization), the executive management subculture (e.g., executive director or primary administrator), and the beneficiary subculture (e.g., beneficiary participant in the shaping of the organization's programs). The functional authority of teachers includes curriculum development, the functional authority of parents includes helping to determine the value and usefulness of the curriculum for their children, and the functional authority of the executive director includes seeing that the curriculum meets local and national standards. Each subculture represents norms and activities that are then derived from those values. Following Glasser (1995), who described the cognition regarding the desire to fulfill fundamental human needs as quality worlds, each subculture, in part, represents the quality worlds implicit in the functions within the organization: teachers prioritize effective pedagogy as part of their quality worlds, parents prioritize their children's educational success as part of their quality worlds, and executive directors prioritize the organization's success as part of their quality worlds.

The fact that there are three spheres and not one internal sphere reflects the point that there are distinctions among the three subcultures, and consequently, developmental tension. The circles within each sphere represent variety or diversity within each sphere. Each subculture represents the values, experiences, and memes or cultural ideas that are brought to the organization by the individuals within each area of function. The areas of overlapping spheres represent points of *informal subcultural partnership* (ISP) where shared values, experiences, and memes strengthen meaning and communication while reinforcing motivation for pursuing the organization's mission. The points of informal subculture partnership also cause diversity to interact. This interaction contributes a variety of cultural ideas (memes) that, if selected for adoption into the subculture, could cause the subculture to evolve. Sometimes the new memes that emerge impact the superordinate culture of the organization.

The overlapping spheres or informal subcultural partnerships are between the expert and executive management, beneficiaries and executive management, and experts and beneficiaries. The intersecting center of the three spheres represents the interconnection of all three subcultures. This center is the nucleus for the organizations' bimodal symmetry. The circling arrows within the three spheres represent collective leadership involving executives, experts, and beneficiaries who lead the subcultures, formally and informally, toward a unified organizational direction.

The overarching circle that subsumes the three interconnected spheres represents the overall culture of the organization. The overall culture of the organization is derived from the collective leadership, the nucleus of informal subculture partnership, and the formal culture of the agency, e.g., cultural artifacts such as the mission statement, bylaws, job descriptions, polices, program descriptions, and procedures.

The formal organizational culture utilizes bureaucratic characteristics to protect the integrity of the mission and to stay within the capacity of the organization. The bureaucratic aspects of the organization are used to express downward power that causes the mission to frame the boundaries of organizational activities while institutionalizing program beneficiary access to developing the quality of the policies and programming. The policies, procedures, and structure then institutionalize the integrity of group decision-making within the organization and help to maintain justice for its program beneficiary base.

Justice is collectively defined through formalized procedures and organizational structure. This process is guided by a clearly defined division of labor, including clarifying scope and limitations of influence within these cross-functional collaborative groups through written job descriptions. These methods establish a consensus model at the decision-making level of the organization as far as the quality of programming is concerned, which in effect institutionalizes a structure that protects and encourages the collective upward expressions of power, as described by Greiner and Schein (1988).

Through protecting group decision-making, particularly as it involves program beneficiaries in shaping the quality of their programs, the structures allow program beneficiaries to exercise upward power that shapes the organizations' policies, goals, and activities to fit the collective needs of the organizations' program beneficiaries within the framework of the mission. Furthermore, through policy and procedure, these organizations establish structure for the expression of sideways power as offered by Greiner and Schein as it relates to maintaining the integrity of the group decision-making process in general.

Therefore the superordinate circle in the graphic, in its totality, represents the common and prioritized informal and formal values and the cultural norms (organizational behavior) that are to some degree sown or dispersed into the external environment of the not-for-profit organization through interacting with beneficiaries, supporters, and interorganizational collaborations as well as through advocacy. These values, cultural norms, and memes influence leaders in the community and consequently other organizations and government institutions in the community of the not-for-profit organization. That is, the external organizations with the most influence over the Healthy (microcultural) Democracy are influenced to be supportive of the HMD organization and sometimes themselves adopt cultural artifacts reflective of memes sown by the influencing HMD.

In between the overarching circle and the interconnected spheres is the area where beneficiary requirements are incorporated in the HMD's programs and high-quality programming is produced. Healthy (microcultural) Democracies, through formal organizational culture and informal cultural partnerships, systematically focus diverse function and quality worlds toward producing the programs of the organization in a manner that continuously enhances usefulness—and value—to the beneficiaries of the organization's mission. This is the essence of Healthy Democracy.

This theory is, of course, based largely on one study. More research is needed, none of which will be more important than participatory evaluation of efforts within grassroots organizations to create

Healthy Democracy.

I have no doubt Healthy Democracy will vary with organization mission, constituency, and size of organization. Nonetheless, the organizational culture outline (the Healthy Democracy model) presented in my findings is a compelling guide. It offers us a reference point to begin our journey to greater democracy in our organizations, and as we shall see in the next chapter, potentially our nation.

CHAPTER **16**

Spreading the Healthy Democracy Meme throughout the Systems of Society

HEALTHY (MICROCULTURAL) DEMOCRACY produces high-quality programs by bringing together the best elements of both the for-profit and not-for-profit worlds. The giving nature of the not-for-profit organization is enhanced by the bottom-line focus that drives continuous improvement and entrepreneurship in the for-profit world. In the not-for-profit sector, the capacity for charity *is* the bottom line. A culture that enhances the scope and impact of charity in such a large and influential sector of society as the not-for-profit is a compelling ideal. One cannot help but wonder about the impact of a not-for-profit sector firmly built on a foundation of Healthy (microcultural) Democracy.

A not-for-profit sector built on effective, efficient, entrepreneurial, ethical, and empathic relationships and focused on program beneficiary requirements would provide society with untold advances. With more research, awareness, and effort, perhaps this wonderful ideal will take root and grow. Perhaps this is already happening and we have yet to sufficiently document the phenomena.

The organizations of my study emerged organically in response to environmental conditions that threatened the propagation of cultural ideas (memes) that their members highly valued. The assumption is that these two organizations are not anomalies, and there are other organizations that have developed similar cultural characteristics over the last half century in the not-for-profit sector.

The preliminary research for suitable subjects to serve as primary case studies for my empirical research (as well as literature review) suggests that a growing number of organizations may be taking on characteristics akin to those identified in the Healthy (microcultural) Democracy model. The conjecture is that HMDs may be influencing cultural changes in their environments at this very moment. They effectively spread new beliefs, assumptions, and norms about how to achieve the objectives of the people these various not-for-profit serve, and these memes at times help shape the organizations in their environment that they interact with.

Healthy (microcultural) Democracies are organizations that exhibit a set of human systems that may, in concert with other such organizations, have the potential to aid the middle and lower classes of the world with survival and reproduction issues. One can imagine these organizations serving as the bricks and mortar for the foundation of a society that realizes democracy's greater potential. Depending on the success of the HMDs, one could even imagine how such organizational culture might provide the impetus for human cultural evolution. According to Richerson and Boyd (2005, 206-207)

> In *On the Origins of Species*, Darwin famously argued that three conditions are necessary for adaptation by natural selection: there must be a "struggle for existence" so that not all individuals survive and reproduce: there must be variation so that some types are more likely to survive and reproduce than others; and variation must be heritable so that the offspring of survivors resemble their parents.
>
> Darwin usually focused on individuals, but the multi-level selection approach tells us that same three postulates apply to *any* reproducing entity—molecules, genes and cultural groups...The only requirement is that there are persistent

cultural differences between groups, and these differences must affect the groups' competitive ability. Winning groups must replace losing groups, but losers need not be killed. The members of losing groups just have to disperse or be assimilated into the victorious group. If losers are resocialized by conformity or punishment, even very high rates of physical migration need not result in the erosion of cultural differences.

Certainly organizational theory scholars have never specifically made the claim that organizational culture (i.e., cultural groups) of the sort proposed has any capacity for affecting the cultural evolution of humanity. However, some organizational theorists have suggested that organizations can affect their environments. Jeffrey Pfeffer (1997, 4) defined organizational theory, in part, as "the mutual effects of environments, including resource and task, political, and cultural environments on organizations and vice versa." Organizations and their environments are interrelated social constructs that influence one another, so this can mean that the reality of a human environment, if viewed as a highly complex organization, can be altered by choice. Hatch (1997, 42) explained social construction theory in this way:

> Since the decision makers, by collecting and analyzing information, create the environment they respond to, we say they socially construct the reality of their environment and enact what they take to be the objective world . . . If organizations are social constructions, then we reconstruct them continuously and could, if we were conscious of these processes, change them in the reconstruction process. Symbolic-interpretive research, in examining the subjective social foundations of organizational realities, begins to make us conscious of our participation in organizational processes. This dawning realization links symbolic-interpretive perspectives with postmodernists who want to take control of these processes and reconstruct the organizational world along more emancipated lines.

According to Hatch, *resource dependence theory* suggests that although organizations tend to be controlled by their environments, they can influence counterdependence in order to establish more self-determination. This view encourages organizations to identify their critical resources and manage their resource dependencies. Hatch (1997, 80) elucidated this concept:

> Managing all kinds of dependencies includes: developing personal relationships with members of firms on which yours is dependent, and establishing formal ties such as taking up membership on their board of directors or inviting one of their officers to sit on your board. In the area of managing regulatory dependencies, a common strategy in the U.S. is to send lobbyists to Washington to influence legislators, for example, to work for competitive trade agreements or to vote for favorable corporate tax laws or government funding of research and development.

The point is that organizations influence their environments. They do this not only through competition, marketing, and advocacy, but also through collaboration and strategic alliances with other organizations (see Hill 2000; McLaughlin 1988; Salamon 1999; Sjostrand 1999). The idea that not-for-profits can influence other organizations is suggested by my empirical research.

Relationships between leaders of organizations key to the success of the Charter School and Advocacy organizations in my study, tended to become more aligned over time with these not-for-profits.

Not-for-profit organizations influence government units. Government influences the business sector (and vice versa). Businesses, through corporate giving, influence not-for-profits. Not-for-profits, governments, and businesses are becoming more and more linked into networks (Dovi 2002; Minkoff 2002; Yankey and Willen 2005). Organizations (e.g., churches, schools, clubs) influence their members as well (Schein 1992). Members of each organization belong to numerous networks of associates, co-workers, friends, and family that, presumably, influence each other. Clearly, through these many networks of interaction, organizations influence their environments and society in general.

From a *network theory* perspective, it could be argued that small organizations in concert with one another can affect the larger environment. Strogatz (2003, 231, 232) explained network theory, also known as *small world theory*:

> Network theory is concerned with the relationships between individuals, the patterns of interactions. The precise nature of the individuals is downplayed, or even suppressed, in hopes of uncovering deeper laws. A network theorist will look at any system of interlinked components and see an abstract pattern of dots connected by lines. It's the pattern that matters, the architecture of relationships, not the identities of the dots themselves. Viewed from these lofty heights, many networks, seemingly unrelated, begin to look the same . . . Our analysis revealed that whether the nodes in the network are neurons or computers, people or power plants, everyone is connected to everyone else by a short chain of intermediaries. In other words, the "small world" phenomenon is much more than a curiosity of human social life: It's a unifying feature of diverse networks found in nature and technology.

It can be argued that network theory is applicable to not-for-profit organizations as well. Furthermore, organizational behavior of one not-for-profit organization can influence others, and this could, theoretically, result in a domino effect on organizational behavior within their networks. These networks in turn could influence other networks of organizations, like government and businesses, resulting in a cascading effect on society.

Strogatz (2003, 265, 266) explored how a small number of members could transform large networks of which they are a part:

All these social phenomena involve herd behavior, where each person relies on the decisions of others to guide his or her own actions. More abstractly, imagine a network of any kind of nodes—companies, people, countries, or other decision makers—and suppose that each node is facing the same binary choice: adopt a new technology or not, riot or not, sign the Kyoto treaty or not. As in Granovetter's model, the decision to adopt, riot, or sign is determined by how many other nodes have already chosen to do so, except that now each node only pays attention to its specific set of "neighbors"—the nodes whose decisions influence it . . . Each node's threshold is defined as the fraction of neighbors who must take action before it will. To allow for diversity in the population, Duncan assumed that some nodes are more adventurous than others, and also that some are better connected . . . Finally, given its allotted number of neighbors, each node forges those links to members of the population chosen at random . . . The game starts when one node is randomly chosen as a seed, an innovator who decided to take the plunge. Visualize it as a domino falling over. Then, one by one, in random order, each node looks at its neighbors and checks what proportion of them have toppled. If its threshold has been transgressed, it tips. Otherwise it stays upright. After each node has taken its turn, the process of checking and toppling begins anew.

Through the lens of network theory, it is clear how organizational culture could emerge in one or a few organizations (microculture) and then move to other similar organizations, and eventually to the larger culture of society (macroculture) depending on its level of success. This opens the possibility that not-for-profit organizations could purposefully spread culture similarly and effect change in the macroculture (memes) of society. Moreover, to surmise that organizations throughout a society can intentionally influence the macroculture of humanity is to suggest that humans can participate in their own cultural evolution. Birch (1972) suggested that Le Conte, who proposed three laws of organic evolution, believed humans do just that when he wrote:

> "Organic evolution," [Le Conte] said "is by pushing upward and onward from below and behind, human process by a drawing upward and onward from above and in front by attractive forces of ideals." Le Conte was convinced that the evolution of human society was a participatory evolution which was determined by the conscious purposes of man. . . Perhaps ten thousand million years ago there was primeval chaos and now here we are, creatures who can consciously determine our own future . . . Man's capacity to make discoveries, then to communicate and to learn, was a new sort of inheritance which made a new sort of evolution possible. To the extent that man can choose goals and discover the means to achieve them, he is in charge of his evolutionary future. That is what cultural evolution implies. Instead of being molded by the forces of the external world we mold the world to suit our purposes. (Dobzhansky 1962; Lerner 1968) . . . The ingredients of conscious participatory evolution are awareness of possibilities not yet realized, a reaching forward with passionate concern to these possibilities and the discovery of ways of making the possible real. The, as yet, unrealized values of the future are a real cause in changing the present.

If the theory that organizations can create counterdependencies in their environments (Hatch 1997; Pfeffer 1997) is accepted, then, in essence, one accepts that organizations can influence their environment. If the theory of Weeks and Gulanic (2003) that organizations are best thought of as cultural identities is accepted, then it is clear how culture spreads from person to person and how the influence of an organization on its environment could be cultural. If it is true that organizations (including not-for-profit organizations) can act like the nodes in a network, as Strogatz (2003) described, then it is not an impossible leap to envision how culture could spread from not-for-profit to not-for-profit. This proliferation of culture could have cascading effects on the culture of organizations, not only within their respective networks, but other organizations throughout the sector and also on the government and business sectors as a result of inter-sector alliances and interactions such as advocacy.

Ultimately, this cascading could influence the macroculture of modern civilization. If Birch (1972) is correct, macrocultural change could progress to the level of cultural evolution; that is, it could influence beliefs and assumptions, values and norms, and cultural artifacts of our nation. Following these theories (Birch 1972; Hatch 1997; Strogatz 2003; Weeks and Galunic 2003), one can easily imagine how the culture of organizations could theoretically affect the cultural evolution of humankind. Since culture is rooted in the values and norms of society, such cultural evolution has implications on how society will use emerging technologies such as genetic manipulation (e.g., the genetic man theory). Culture affects not only the thinking and actions of humanity, it affects how we use our technology to respond to the disasters purportedly facing humanity today.

The suggestion here is that, as the first developmental stage, mimetic institutional pressures cascade into normative institutional pressures. These in turn inspire coercive institutional pressures, and the organizations of society are moved toward a more citizen-focused model in order to achieve social legitimacy. The result would likely be a more deliberative democracy (see Hill 2000) through some form of civic republicanism (see Barber 1984; Etzioni 1993; Hill 2000).

In short, a not-for-profit sector comprising a large number of Healthy (microcultural) Democracies (e.g., 20/80 rule) could be positioned to help establish a macroculture that functions like an evolutionarily stable strategy (ESS) for the middle and underclasses of society worldwide. ESS is " . . . a strategy that if most members of a population adopt, cannot be bettered by an alternative strategy" (Dawkins 1989). This macroculture would stress mutualism and promote collaboration and functional authority, high ethical standards including hard work and fortitude, social entrepreneurship with individual and social responsibility, performance management, servant leadership, forgiveness with clear limitations, and identification or empathy across a great diversity of humanity. These norms would help to establish a *citizen*-focused partnership quality culture *society* or, for simplicity's sake, a *Healthy (macrocultural)* Democracy (HD). It would help form a more citizen-focused civilization that is also more efficient and effective at solving the many problems of humanity.

Below is a graphic that illustrates this theory.

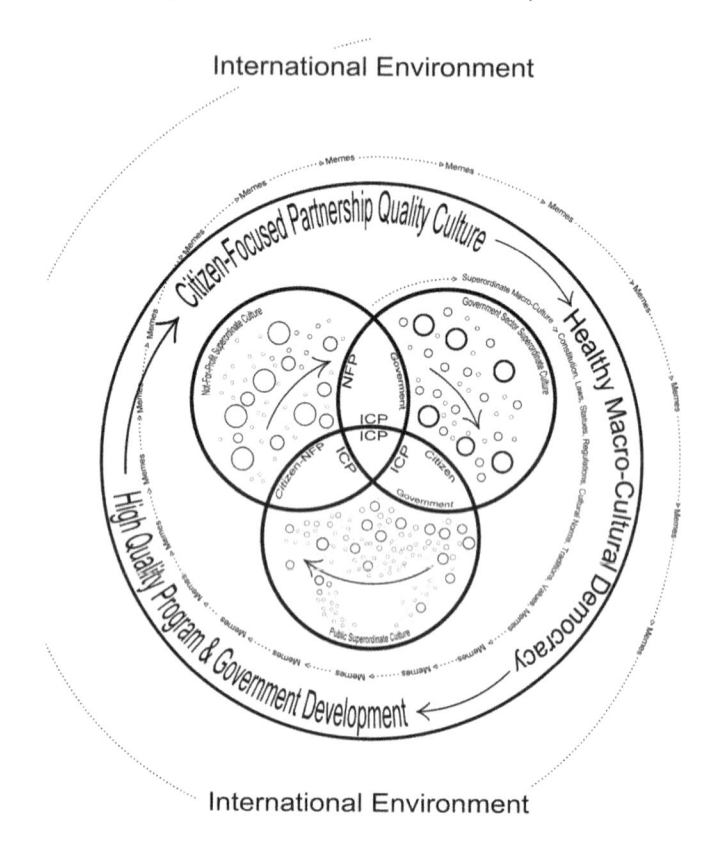

FIGURE 2. International environment.

Spreading the Healthy Democracy Meme throughout the Systems of Society

The three interconnected spheres in Figure 2 represent different overarching cultures within the broader society of a Healthy (macrocultural) Democracy, or Healthy Democracy (HD) for short. Each sphere also represents a variety of functional authority, expertise, and a wide variety of missions or focuses. Specifically, these cultures are the not-for-profit sector overarching culture, the government sector overarching culture, and the overarching culture of the public relative to the other two sectors. In other words, the final sphere reflects the public's values, worldviews, traditions, and norms pertinent to both the not-for-profit and government sectors activities.

The circles within the government sphere represent different local, regional, and federal government units. The circle within the not-for-profit sphere represent the not-for-profit communities of organizations (e.g., alliances, functional and subfunctional areas, geographic groupings), and the circles within the public sphere represent individual citizens. The reader will note that for-profit corporations are not apparent in this graphic. In the Healthy Democracy (HD) model, the owners, stockholders and employees of corporations are included in the public sphere as individual citizens, but without any greater influence than any other citizen. They like all citizens would have access to not-for-profit and government representation. This arrangement would of course require the barring of major donations to politicians running for office and likely some form of public financing of elections as well. Healthy Democracy isn't subservient to the loudest or most powerful voice(s) but rather uses structure to focus decision-making on shaping the commons through the process of collectively defined justice in order to serve all the people in equitable ways. A Healthy Democracy would be concerned with participation in high-quality (Cox, 1999) programs and government development for the benefit of the citizens, as the overall citizen body shapes it, as opposed to how dominant citizens or major corporations would shape output through donations.

Within each sphere, Healthy (microcultural) Democracy (HMD) is at work. Not only does the not-for-profit sector involve citizens in shaping policy of individual organizations, but government and large corporate institutions are structured so that the spirit of Healthy (microcultural) Democracy shapes the process of decision-making. For example, large corporations would involve customers and citizen stakeholders through democratized structures and processes for shaping not only products but also policy when it affects the commons.

The arrows within the three spheres have dual representations: (a) the spreading of Healthy Democracy (influence and memes) between the not-for-profit, citizen, and government sectors in order to bring them together in partnership and (b) the collective leadership (public, not-for-profit, and government) of the nation for unity and common direction—that direction, in part, being a Healthy (macrocultural) Democracy.

As in Figure 1 (Healthy microcultural Democracy), the HD graphic shows the overlapping spheres indicating *informal cultural partnership* (ICP), this time between the overarching sector cultures. Similarly, the center intersection of all three spheres represents the intersection of all three overarching sector cultures. This intersecting of culture forms the nucleus for the bimodal symmetry of the nation. The larger globe represents the macroculture of the nation. The macroculture includes the informal culture (e.g., personal cultures, values and norms, traditions) and the formal cultures of the nation (e.g., its constitution, laws, statues, regulations). Like the HMD, the Healthy Democracy (HD) of a nation would institutionalize downward power to assure a mission—Constitution, Bill of Rights-driven process and operation within the capacity of the organization or government. It would also institutionalize upward as well as sideways power. The macroculture would tend to influence other nations via its citizens, foreign support efforts, diplomacy, and international collaborations (e.g., trade, hunger relief, and international regulation).

In between the three sector spheres and the macroculture (represented by the overarching circle) of the nation are various not-for-profit, government, and private citizen partnerships that produce high-quality enterprises for the benefit of the citizen body. The citizen-focused partnership process would function similarly to beneficiary-focused partnership process for program development in the Healthy (microcultural) Democracy within not-for-profits.

If the problems facing humanity today are rooted in human culture, then what we may need is a new overarching culture—one that transcends race, class, and religion and is focused on solving the problems of the citizens of the nation through collaboration—a culture that encourages a more reciprocal, altruistic version of ourselves. We may need to evolve beyond the culture of greed and zero-sum fixation, not only for altruistic reasons but also as a matter of self-interest. Healthy (macrocultural) Democracy has the potential to help us achieve this goal.

The Healthy (macrocultural) Democracy model is, of course, theoretical. As a society, we are a long way from this type of civilization. To be clear, the suggestion at the time this book is being written is not that the not-for-profit sector has the critical mass of Healthy (microcultural) Democracies to begin the cascading influence, but rather that this could change. Furthermore, it may be changing at this very moment. Two hundred years ago, it was almost inconceivable that the United States could be free of slavery or that women would have the right to vote. Yet the idea of enslaving all Americans of African descent and barring all women from voting is today the inconceivable. Evil institutions of our past have been changed, in large part, as a matter of our nation's evolution and survival. What is being suggested is that human culture evolves, and humanity may have the burgeoning organizational theory and will to build a more reciprocal, altruistic civilization. Moreover, humanity might build a more efficient, effective, social-entrepreneurial, ethical, and empathetic democratic world if it were a matter of survival—and quite possibly it is.

By becoming conscious of Healthy (microcultural) Democracy and the theoretical potential for Healthy (macrocultural) Democracy to emerge as a result, we can mindfully participate in cultural evolution in the direction of greater democracy by developing our organizations based on the HMD model. Those organizations that do this should develop a stronger, more active base of support and consequently, pound for pound, should outperform the average not-for-profit that does not adopt some adaptation of HMD. If we consider Axelrod's Prisoner's Dilemma experiments, the HMD organization, in concert with other similar organizations (i.e., those that choose "cooperate"), should, in time, theoretically outperform the organizations based on war culture, that is, zero-sum hierarchies that choose "defect."

Through our efforts to change our grassroots organizations (along with being socially responsible as individuals and passively resisting oligarchy), we could help to initiate a domino effect on the macroculture of society by encouraging the organizations of society to move toward a Healthy Democracy model in order to achieve social legitimacy. In this way we can establish a new environment that encourages a more reciprocal, altruistic biology of human behavior—a socialization process focused on the many, by the many, and for the many.

CHAPTER 17

Tomorrow Morning

PETER DRUCKER (1990, 49) has said,

> We are creating tomorrow's society of citizens through the nonprofit service institution. And in that society, everybody is a leader, everybody is responsible, everybody acts. Everybody focuses himself or herself. Everybody raises the vision, the competence, and the performance of his or her organization. Therefore, mission and leadership are not just things to read about, to listen to. They are things to do something about. Things that you can, and should, convert from good intentions and from knowledge into effective action, not next year, but tomorrow morning.

It doesn't matter where we stand on the many wedge issues that are promoted within our society. Human beings will always disagree. What matters most is how we approach our disagreements, and Healthy Democracy offers us a constructive approach to pursuing our divergent goals and approaching conflicts within the internal and external environments in a constructive manner. It offers us a blueprint for a healthy people-focused society. Healthy Democracy will strengthen the pursuit of our organizations' missions by strengthening our organizations and potentially our network cultures.

The movement for Healthy Democracy will be long and arduous. It took some fifty years of strategic action on the behalf of the Few to create the Trump–Pence reality we now live in. It will take time for our cultural evolution within our political revolution to evolve. In the meantime, our organizations will learn to build community internally. Each movement will learn to effectively collaborate and respect diversity within its own movement as a precursor to collaborating and respecting the diversity in sister movements.

Ultimately, the experience of being a Healthy Democracy will teach us to collaborate and respect the diversity even within countermovements to our own because even adversaries can be allies at times. For example, on the issue of media reform, advocacy groups as divergent as gun rights and peace activists have been allies.

It doesn't matter if your work is in the arts or in athletics, social service, advocacy, research, or religion—I believe the Healthy Democracy model can help your cause. So if you are active in the not-for-profit sector, do what you have been doing, but do it more effectively, efficiently, entrepreneurially, ethically, and empathetically. Involve those you profess will benefit from the mission of your organization.

Now, more than ever, is the time to organize your personal life, and organize your group, not-for-profit, or community. The 2016 election changed many things, but not our potential. There is no policy achievement of the Trump–Pence reality (or the oligarchy of billionaires that they represent) that can't be countered and eventually undone. But first we must shine light on what is lurking in the shadows beneath Trump–Pence's media-splashing actions and how they are being used as cover as this administration usurps the resources of our nation and the structures of our democracy.

When I was a young man, I witnessed (in city politics) events that (in all but outcome) parallel the 2016 presidential election. I was involved in a cutting-edge program to address racism in a city. The city was essentially a one-political-party town. This effort was spearheaded by a not-for-profit organization chaired by the mayor of that city, who happened to be an African American. The executive director of the organization was also black. When committees of this organization, comprising ordinary citizens of all races and religions, began proposing revolutionary change, there was an attempt (as I saw it) by certain elements of the power structure to infiltrate and install within this organization a leadership more likely to pursue goals that maintained the status quo of racial inequity in that city. When this failed, these elements advocated for the mayor to step in and help them realize their leadership desires for this organization. The mayor refused. Soon afterwards, elements within the political party that the mayor belonged to organized against that mayor in the next election. Coincidence? In retrospect, the opposition selected (who was white) to run against the mayor made it look a lot like they had taken their strategies right out of the Trump playbook. Through media complicity (with little campaign spending), the opposition to the mayor used images of police and African Americans in conflict and also allegations of corruption and conspiracy, apparently calculated to divide the voters along racial lines. It was working. It looked like the mayor would lose the election. But at the last minute, some key supporters of the mayor were able to successfully expose this tactic for what it was—a divide-and-conquer strategy devised to manipulate whites into voting for whites and blacks into voting for blacks (irrespective of their best interest), and this would certainly defeat the black mayor in a town where the majority was white. The mayor won re-election.

If we make our cultural evolution in our political revolution about whites vs. people of color, we will lose. If we make it about women vs. men or right vs. left, we will lose. Even if we make this cultural evolution about rich vs. poor, we will lose. We are weaker when we are against each other and stronger when we are for boundary-expanding[10] ideas such as Healthy Democracy. Therefore, this cultural evolution in our political revolution cannot be just a battle against,

---

10   According to Kirby (2006) Boundary spanning people, ideas, places and cultural artifacts connect and focus the diverse interests of individuals and consequently help establish successful collaboration.

but rather, more emphatically, a battle *for*. *This battle is for democracy*—not what side of our divisions will prevail on the wedge issues, but instead how we will responsibly address the divisions that we will always have. A major political party could possibly be the conduit for this movement, but it would require groups of Healthy Democracy advocates that would form a powerful wing of the major political party. This wing would be committed to the ideals of Healthy Democracy first and the political party second. Its objective would be to transform the power centers of the party into bastions of servant leaders intent on restructuring the party to align it with values, norms, and cultural artifacts consistent with Healthy Democracy. But this can only come about from external movements pressuring a major political party to open the door and allow people representing the Healthy Democracy wing to enter.

With or without one of the two major parties that control our political system, we have the potential to move forward with creating our own reality, and that reality can be Healthy Democracy—if we so choose. It is a reality we can spread by modeling the behaviors that exemplify it in our daily activities and in the organizations under our control. But it will take time. This battle begins in our hearts and minds and deeds, extends to our families, friends, schools, grassroots organizations, religious centers, and advocacy groups. It is a battle for the soul of all American institutions because it is a battle for the soul of America.

As imperfect as it was, we have lost the precious little democracy we once had. Our representatives no longer represent the middle class at all, nor do they fully enforce the people's constitutional rights. There is a battle to return to the American tradition of government afforded by our constitutional democratic republic of earlier times that was at least more attentive to the requirements of white middle class males. This battle cry comes from elements deep within a new conservative populism.

There is also a growing awareness that we have never truly had a government based on the belief "it is self-evident that all [humans] are created equal," and therefore we have never in fact had a true democracy. Authentic democracy is a quest championed by American progressivism.

Elements from both the right and the left are headed in the same direction—greater democracy than we have now! But both movements have been co-opted. When we free our minds, we will free our movements from the parasites that co-opt our hearts and therefore control our minds. Then we will be on the march. We, the people, will be marching toward greater democracy, but from different perspectives. The questions are: Can we free these movements from co-option? If one leg of these parallel movements frees itself from co-option, can it drag the other until it gains its freedom? Will we coordinate the left and right movements toward greater democracy enough to carry us successfully to this end, or will we allow co-option of these divergent movements to cause the people to stumble over themselves and fall to bitter defeat?

We see the barriers wedged between us play out often in our media. Instead of focusing on common goals our consciousness are directed toward our divisions. Instead of facilitating how we might best bridge our differences on wedge issues, prioritizing win–win solutions when possible (compromise when necessary), our leaders are limited to starkly choosing sides. They are required to be zero-sum, us against them. They must be for abortion or against it, for guns or against them, for more taxes or less taxes, for affirmative action or not, for gay marriage or against it—they are required to be zero-sum oriented! Consequently, they encounter a stumbling block that impedes our quest for Healthy Democracy. Depending on how they answer, there is a target that the media (interviewer) will have successfully placed on their backs. If the facilitator (would-be leader) answers that they support the conservative view of a wedge issue, then the target that attracts the ammunition of progressives will be placed on their backs. If they choose the progressive position on a wedge issue, the questioner will have placed the target that draws the attacks from conservatives. If their answer is eclectic (the greatest sin of all), they get both targets placed on their backs.

The point is this: the media will have successfully shut down the connection between the would-be facilitator (leader) and the minds of some segment of the population, thereby disabling a bridge to Healthy Democracy. This segment will no longer hear what the facilitator says, because the rational mind is shut down and the emotional mind is activated and in control. We shift our consciousness from pursuing win–win solutions to zero-sum outcomes. Resentment, disdain, even hate fills the soul when the rational mind is disengaged under these conditions. Our minds, in a sense, fall under the control of those who can place these targets on the backs of our would-be facilitative leaders. If this is not mind control, what is it? If we want a Healthy Democracy, we first must defeat those techniques that control our minds. Healthy Democracy requires free minds. The point is not that we disagree on the wedge issues. Of course we disagree; that is why we need a democracy to address our governance. The solution to our wedge issues is not found in the positions we take with respect to them, but how we respond to the disagreements we will always have, and that is the hope and potential of Healthy Democracy.

At the heart of the American experiment lie two essential worldviews that animate all democratic republics—conservatism and progressivism—the values of stability vs. change. Change without stability is chaos. Stability without change is stagnation. Change is most constructive with the efficiency of stability at its disposal, and all things are more stable when they can effectively respond to change.

Change and stability are the left and right legs of democracy. Together they perpetuate our ongoing journey to the condition of being of, by, and for all the people equitably. But powerful elements in our society have set them against each other and disabled our democratic republic. When we the people realize the value of both, we will stand straight and carry on to our greater destiny. I believe we can achieve this realization: one person, one family, one organization, one local, city, state, and national government at a time. But the first step must begin with you.

References

Alexander, S. 2006. "Empathy: Sermon XI in the Year-Long Series Twelve Gates to the City: A Spiritual Guide for Full Religious Living." Sermon, May 14, 2006. Bethesda, MD: River Road Unitarian Church.

Axelrod, N. R. 2005. "Board and Leadership Development." In *The Jossey-Bass Handbook of Nonprofit Leadership and Management*, 2nd ed., edited by R. D. Herman, 131-152. San Francisco: Jossey-Bass.

Barbuda, Jr., J. E., and D. W. Wheeler. 2002, rev. 2007. *Becoming a Servant Leader: Do You Have What It Takes?* Lincoln: University of Nebraska-Lincoln, Institute of Agriculture and Natural Resources, Cooperative ExtensionNebGuide. http://extensionpublications.unl.edu/assets/pdf/g1481.pdf

BBC News. 2014. "Study: US Is an Oligarchy, Not a Democracy." April 17, 2014. http://www.bbc.com/news/blogs-echochambers-27074746

Bernays, E. 1928. *Propaganda*. Whale.to./b/bernayspdf

Birch, C. 1972. "Participatory Evolution: The Drive of Creation." *Journal of American Academy of Religion*, Volume XL, Issue 1, June. Pages 147-163

Boggs, W. B. 2004. "TQM and Organizational Culture: A Case Study." *Quality Management Journal* 11, no. 2, 42-52.

Booth, J. 2017. "Islam and Lust." http://classroom.synonym.com/islam-lust-12086653.html

Borg, M. 1997. *Jesus and Buddha: The Parallel Sayings*. Berkeley, California: Seastone Publishing.

Burke, J. 2006. "The United States Is Ill-Prepared to Wage a New Cold War." *Eurasia Insights*, May 8, 2006. http://www.eurasianet.org/department/insight/ articale s/eav050806.shtml

Burton, J. W. 1990. *Conflict Resolution: Towards Problem Solving.* http://gmu.edu/academic/pcs/burton.html.

Campbell, T. C. 2006. *The China Study*. Dallas, TX: BenBella Books, Inc.

Catechism of the Catholic Church. 1995. New York: Doubleday.

Cha, A.E. 2017. First Human Embryo Editing Experiment in U.S. "Corrects" Genes for Heart Condition. *Washington Post*. http://washingtonpost.com/news/to-your-healthy/wp/2017/08/02/first-human-embryo-editing-experiment-in-u-s-corrects-gene-for-heart-condition/?utm_term=.lab659b58855

Christakis, N. A., and J. H. Fowler. 2009. *Connected*. New York: Simon and Schuster, Inc.

Collins Dictionary, s.v. "Clarion Call." Accessed June 6, 2019.

Confessore, N. 2003. "Welcome to the Machine: How The GOP Disciplined K Street and Made Bush Supreme." https://washingtonmontly.com/magazine/julyaugust-2003/welcome-to-the-machine/

Covey, S. R. 2013. "How to Develop Your Personal Mission Statement." Grand Harbor Press.

Covey, S. R. 2012. "How to Develop Your Family Mission Statement." Simon and Schuster Audio.

Cox, R. O. 1999. "Quality in Nonprofits: No Longer Uncharted Territory." *Quality Progress*, 57-66

Cross, J. C. 1997. *Developing NGOs, the State and Neo-Liberalism: Competition, Partnership or Co-Conspiracy.* Cairo: Department of Sociology, The American University in Cairo.

Curran, C. J. 2005. "Organizational Culture: The Path to Better Organization." *Journal for Nonprofit Management* 9, no. 1, 28-40.

Dale, C. 2009. *The Subtle Body: An Encyclopedia of Your Energetic Anatomy*. Boulder, CO: Sounds True, Inc.

Dawkins, R. 1989. *The Selfish Gene*. New York: Oxford University Press.

References

Deen Show, N.D. https://www.thedeenshow.com

Deming, W. E. 1990. *Out of the Crisis*. Cambridge, MA: MIT Press.

Diamond, J. 2005. *Collapse: How Societies Choose to Fail or Succeed*. New York: Penguin Books.

Dictionary.com, s.v., "balance," accessed November 7, 2013.

Dictionary.com, s.v., "corporate," accessed December 1, 2016.

Dictionary.com, s.v., "faith," accessed September 9, 2017.

Dictionary.com, s.v., "passive resistance," accessed February 4, 2015.

Dovi, S. "A Democratic Ethics of International Advocacy." Paper presented at the annual meeting of the American Political Science Association, Boston, MA, August 2002.

Drucker, Peter. 1990. *Managing the Non-Profit Organizations*: Principles and Practice. New York, NY: HarperCollins Publishers.

The Economist. 2016. "Free Speech Under Attack." June 4, 2016. https://www.economists.com/news/leaders/2169909-curbs-free-speech-are-growing-tighter-it-time-speak-out-under-attack

Education Commission of the States. 2005. http://www.ecs.org/charter-schools-policies/

Emoto, M., 2005. *The Hidden Messages In Water*. New York: Atria Books

Eschner, Kat. 2018. "CRISPR Has Many Promising Applications-But The Gene-Edited Twins Represent Something More Troubling." http://www.popsci.com/crispr-gene-editing-babies-safety

Firth, N. 2010. "The 'Violent' Gene: Genetic Mutation Found Only in Finnish Men that Makes Them Fight." http://www.dailymail.co.uk/sciencetech/article.1341100/theviolentgene

Foley, M., and B. Edwards. 2002. "How Do Members Count? Membership, Governance, and Advocacy in the Nonprofit World." In *Exploring Organizations and Advocacy: Governance And Accountability*, edited by M. Montilla and E. Reid. Washington, DC: Urban Institute Press.

Fuhrman, J. 2017. *Fast Food Genocide*. San Francisco: HarperOne.

Galbraith, J. K. 1983. *The Anatomy of Power*. Boston: Houghton Mifflin Company

Glasser, W. 1995. *The Control Theory Manager: Combining the Control Theory of William Glasser with the Wisdom of W. Edwards Deming to Explain What Is Quality*. New York: Harper Perennial.

Golden Rule—Langley Baha'i Community. Retrieved 2020 from https://www.langleybahai.org>golden-rule.html

Greenleaf, R. 1970. *The Servant as Leader*. Westfield, IN: Greenleaf Center for Servant Leadership.

Greiner, L. E., and V. E. Schein. 1988. *Power and Organization Development: Mobilizing Power to Implement Change*. Reading, MA: Addison-Wesley.

Haidt, J. 2012. *The Rightous Mind: Why Good People are Divided by Politics and Religion*. New York: Pantheon

Hall, P. D. 2005. "Historical Perspectives on Nonprofit Organizations in the United States." In *Jossey-Bass Handbook of Nonprofit Leadership and Management*, edited by R.D. Herman. San Francisco: Jossey-Bass.

Hannan, M. T., and J. Freeman. 1989. *Organizational Ecology*. Cambridge, MA: Harvard University Press.

Hatch, M. J. 1997. *Organization Theory: Modern, Symbolic and Postmodern Perspectives*. New York: Oxford University Press

Hayden, T. 2002. "A Theory Evolves: How Evolution Really Works, and Why It Matters More Than Ever." *U.S. News and World Report* 133, no. 4, 42-6, 48, 50.

Hayden, R. 2002. "Dictators of Virtue? States, NGOs, and the Imposition of Democratic Values." *Harvard International Review*, 56-61.

Hertbert, N. 1987. *Quantum Reality: Beyond the New Physics*. New York: Anchor Books

Hill, Frances R. 2000. *Nonprofit Organizations' Advocacy Activities: Association, Participation and Representation*. Washington, DC: Urban Institute Press.

Hudson, F. M. 2001. "Life Launch: A Passionate Guide to the Rest of Your Life." The Hudson Institute Press.

Hudson Institute of Santa Barbara, 2000. "Planning for Change." The Hudson Institute of Santa Barbara

Islam.ru. Retrieved 2/25/2020. www.islam.ru/en/content/story/golden-rule-islam

Jenny, H. [1967] 1974. *Cymatics: A Study of Wave Phenomena and Vibration*, vol. I and II. Moroskop.org

Joad, G., and Randall, K., 2019. *Policing Violence the Sixth Leading Cause of Death for Youngmen in the U.S.* International Committee of the Fourth International

Jones, S., Brush, K., Baily, S., McInye, J. Kahn, J., Nelson, B., Stickle, L. 2017. *Navigating SEL From the Inside Out: Looking Inside and Across 25 Leading SEL Programs: A Practical Resource for Schools and OST Providers. Harvard Graduate School*. Massachusetts.

Jordan, C., J. Orozco, and A. Averett. 2001. *Emerging Issues in School, Family, and Community Connections*. Austin, TX: National Center for Family and Community Connections with Schools, Southwest Education Development Laboratory.

Kendall, J. 2002. "How Child Abuse and Neglect Damage the Brain." *The Boston Globe*.

Kennerly, M. S. 2010. "eBay v. Newmark: Al Franken Was Right, Corporations Are Legally Required to Maximize Profits." https://www.litigationandtrial.com/2010/09/articles/series/special-comment/ebay-v-newmark-al-franken-was-right-corporations-are-legally-required-to-maximize-profits/

Kirby, K. E. 2006. *The Use of Boundary Objects for Purposeful Change in Higher Education*. Philadelphia: University of Pennsylvania.

Klein, N. 2007. *The Shock Doctrine*: Gordonsville, VA: Holtzbrinck Publishers, LLC.

Kraus, M. W., and P. K. Piff. 2011. *Social Class as Culture: The Convergence of Resources and Rank in the Social Realm*. Association for Psychological Science.

Krugman, H. 1971. "Brain Waves Measure of Media Involvement." *Journal of Advertising*.

Kujala, K., and P. Lillrank, P. 2004. *Total Quality Management as a Cultural Phenomenon*. Helsinki: Helsinki University of Technology.

Kushi, M. 1979. *The Book of Do-In*. Tokyo: Japan Publications.

La Piana, D. 1999. *The Partnership Matrix.* http://www.lapaiana.org/defined/matrix.html.

Light, P.C. 2006. "Searching for Social Entrepreneurs: Who They Might Be, Where They Might Be Found, What They Do." ARNOVA Occasional Paper Series 1, no. 3, 13-38.

Lindstrom, M. 2008. *Buy-ology.* New York: Random House.

Loya, J. A., H. Wan-Li, and J. Chang-Shin. 1998. *The Tao of Jesus: An Experiment in Inter-Traditional Understanding.* New York: Paulist Press.

Lytle, M., 2013. *Body pH: Acid-base Balance and Alkaline Diet.* https://invitehealth.com/article-body-ph-acid-base-balance-and-alkaline-diet.html

McDougall, J. A., and M. McDougall. 2012. *The Starch Solution: Eat the Foods You Love, Regain Your Health and Lose the Weight for Good.* Emmaus, PA: Rodale Publishing.

Mills, D. G. 2004. *It's the Corporate State, Stupid.* http://www.informationclearinghouse.info/article7260.htm

Minkoff, D. C. 2002. "Walking a Political Tightrope: Responsiveness and Internal Accountability in Social Movement Organizations." In *Exploring Organizations and Advocacy: Governance and Accountability,* edited by E. Reid and M. Montilla, 33-48. Washington DC: The Urban Institute.

Nordenstrom, B. E. W. 1983. *Biologically Closed Electric Circuits.* Skarpnack, Sweden: Nordic Medical Publications.

Perlmutter, D. 2013. *Grain Brain: The Surprising Truth About Wheat, Carbs and Sugar—Your Brain's Silent Killer.* New York: Hachette Book Group.

Perry, P. "Scientists Discover How to Implant False Memories." Accessed Bigthink.com.

Perret, R. W. 1998. *Hindu Ethics.* Honolulu: University of Hawaii Press.

Pfeffer, J. 1997. *New Directions for Organization Theory: Problems and Prospects.* Oxford University Press.

Pfeffer, J., and G. R. Salancik. 1978. *The External Control of Organizations: A Resource Dependent Perspective.* New York: Harper and Row.

Phillips, P. and Osborne, B. 2013. Financial Core of the Transnational Corporate Class. *Project Censored: Fearless Speech in Fateful Times*. 2014. projectcensored.org

Pollins, R. 2000. "Anatomy of Clintonomics." *New Left Review* 3. http://newleftreview.org/?page=article&andview=2243

Powell, W. W., and R. Steinberg. 2006. *The Nonprofit Sector: A Research Handbook*. New Haven: Yale University Press.

Pyles, L. 2003. *Transforming the Culture of Advocacy for Social and Economic Justice*. http://www.artesana.com /articles/transforming_culture_advocacy.htm

Racine, E. 2003. "Discourse Ethics as a Ethics of Responsibility: Comparison and Evaluation of Citizen Involvement in Population Genomics." pp 390-397. *The Journal of Law, Medicine and Ethics*.

Rahhal, N. 2019. *Chinese Scientists Who Edited Genes of Twin Girls May Have Supercharged Their Brains Too, Experts Say*. www.Dailymail.com

Rex Research Group. (Retrieved, 2016) "Russian DNA Research." http://www.rexresearch.com/gajarev/gajarev.htm

Richards, C. and L. Martin. 2012. *Epigenetics for Behavioral Ecologists*. Tampa: University of South Florida.

Richerson, P. J., and R. Boyd. 2005. *Not by Genes Alone: How Culture Transformed Human Evolution*. Chicago: University of Chicago.

Robbins, S. P. 1998. *Organizational Behavior: Concepts, Controversies, Applications*. Upper Saddle River, NJ: Prentice Hall.

Russo, A. 2005. *Freedom to Fascism*. Los Angeles: All Your Freedoms, Inc.

Salamon, L. M., H. Anheier, R. List, S. Toepler, S. Sokolowski, and associates. 1999. *Global Civil Society: Dimensions of the Nonprofit Sector*. Baltimore, MD: John Hopkins Center for Civil Society Studies.

Sapolsky, R. (2005. *Biology and Human Behavior: The Neurological Origins of Individuality*, 2nd ed. Chantilly, VA: Teaching Company.

Schaefer, U. 1994. "Ethics for a Global Society." *Baha'i Studies Reviews* 4.1.

Schalch, N. 2006. "1981 Strike Leaves Legacy for American Workers." http//www.npr.org/templates/storyId=5604656

Schein, E. H. 1992. *Organizational Culture and Leadership*. San Francisco: Jossey-Bass.

Schimmel, S. 1997. *The Seven Deadly Sins: Jewish, Christian, and Classical Reflections of Human Psychology*. New York: Oxford University Press.

Sjostrand, S. E. 1999. *The Organization of Non-Profit Activities*. Stockholm, Sweden: Stockholm School of Economics.

Smith, J. M. 2003. *Seeds of Deception*. Fairfield, IA: Yes! Books

Smith, R. S. 2005. *Managing the Challenge of Government Contracts: Handbook of Nonprofit Leadership and Management*, 2nd ed. San Francisco: Jossey-Bass.

Smith, W. C. 1991. *The Meaning and End of Religion*. Fortress Press. Minneapolis

Strogatz, S. 2003. *Sync: The Universe, Nature, and Daily Life*. New York: Theia.

Stull, M. G. 2005. *Intrapreneurship in Nonprofit Organizations: Examining the Factors that Facilitate Entrepreneurial Behavior Among Employees*. Cleveland, OH: Case Western Reserve University.

Vohs, K. D., 2009. "Self-Affirmation and Self-Control: Affirming Core Values Counteracts Ego Depletion." *Journal of Personality and Social Psychology* 96, no. 4, 770.

Walker, J. J. 2006. *The Servant-Led Institution: A Case Study Defining Servant Leadership in the Not-For-Profit Social Organization*. Virginia Beach, VA: Regent University.

Weeks, J., and C. Galunic. 2003. "A Theory of the Cultural Evolution of the Firm: The Intra-Organizational Ecology of Memes." *Organizational Studies* 24, 1309-1352.

Wells, S. D. 2014. "70,000 Food Additives Approved by the FDA – What You Don't Know Will Hurt You." https://www.naturalnews.com/045739_food_additives_FDA_toxic_chemicals.html

Wenk, Gary L., 2010. *How Does Food Affect Our Brain? Our Brains Reward Us For Eating Sugar, Fat and Salt*. Psychologytoday.com

Wikipedia, s.v. "Post WWII economic expansion." Accessed September 24, 2012.

Wikipedia, s.v. "propaganda." Accessed December 6, 2012.

Wikipedia, s.v. "social responsibility." Accessed February 4, 2015.

Wikipedia, s.v. "Dutch East Indian Company." Accessed October 7, 2012.

Worthington, E. L. 2004. *The New Science of Forgiveness*. Greater Good Magazine, UC Berkeley

Yankey, J. A., and C. K. Willen. 2005. "Strategic Alliances." In *The Jossey-Bass Handbook of Nonprofit Leadership and Management*, 2nd ed., edited by R. D. Herman, 254-275. San Francisco: Jossey-Bass.

Bibliography

Abzug, R., and J. S. Simonoff. 2004. *Nonprofit Trusteeship in Different Contexts*. Aldershot, UK: Ashgate.

Alinsky, S. 1946. *Reveille for Radicals*. New York: Vintage Press.

Alinsky, S. 1971. *Rules for Radicals*. New York: Vintage Press.

Arms Control Association. n.d. "Russian Officials Deny Claims of Missing Nuclear Weapons." http://www.armscontrol.org/print/250

Armstrong, K. M. 2003. *There Is No Back Seat Here: A Narrative Case Study of What Influences Parent Stakeholder Participation on a School Engaged on Educational Reform*. Santa Barbara, CA: Fielding Institute.

Babbage, C. 1832. *On the Economy of Machinery and Manufactures*. London: R. Clay, Bread Street Hill.

Baldas, T. 2005. "Tension Grows over Genetic Testing of Employees: Privacy, Potential Discrimination Are Major Concerns." *The National Law Journal*. http://www.law.com/jsp/article.jsp?id=1130499505655

Bamford, J. 2008. *The Shadow Factory: The Ultra-Secret NSA from 9/11 to the Eavesdropping on America*. New York: Random House.

Barnard, C. [1938] 1968. *The Functions of the Executive*. London: Oxford University Press.

BBC News Channel. 2006. "Zimbabwe Faces AIDS Drug Shortage." May 3, 2006. http://news.bbc.co.uk/1/hi/world/africa/4969228.stm

Begley, S. 2008. "Mind Reading Is Now Possible." *Newsweek*, January 21, 2008. http://www.newsweekmagazine.com/id/91688

Bolman, L. G., and T. E. Deal. 2003. *Reframing Organizations: Artistry, Choice, and Leadership*, 3d ed. San Francisco: Jossey-Bass.

Bond, M. H. 1998. *"Unity in Diversity Orientations and Strategies for Building a Harmonious Multicultural Society."* Keynote address presented to the Conference on Multiculturalism: Diversity in Action, Tartu, Estonia. http://bahai-library.com

Bouteneff, M. C. 2006. *Ethical Dimensions of Work-Related Issues Faced by Public-School Principals and Resources to Help Them Resolve These Issues.* NY: Columbia University.

Broom, M. F., and D. C. Klein. 1999. *Power: The Infinite Game.* Ellicott City, MD: Sea Otter Press.

Brown, R. 2004. *School Culture and Organization: Lessons from Research and Experience.* Denver, CO: The Denver Commission on Secondary School Reform.

Bruce, A., and K. Langdon. 2000. *Project Management.* New York: Dorling Kindersley.

Brudney, J. L. 2005. "Designing and Managing Volunteer Programs." In *The Jossey-Bass Handbook of Nonprofit Leadership and Management,* 2nd ed., edited by R. D. Herman, 310-345. San Francisco: Jossey-Bass.

Bruner, R. F., M. R. Eaker, R. E. Freeman, R. E. Spekman, E. O. Teisberg, and S. Venkataraman. 2003. *The Portable MBA,* 4th ed. Hoboken, NJ: John Wiley and Sons.

Burns, J. M. 1963. *The Deadlock of Democracy.* Englewood Cliffs, NJ: Prentice-Hall.

Burns, J. M. 2004. "Moral Leadership and Business Ethics." In *Ethics, The Heart of Leadership,* edited by J. Ciulla. Westport, CT: Prager.

Calhoun, J. M. "An Introduction to Baldrige Basics and the Benefits of Using the Baldrige Criteria to Assess the Performance of Your Organization." Paper presented at the 24th Annual Spring Conference, Teams in the Workplace, Gaithersburg, MD, March 2002.

Campbell, R. 1998. "Innovative Community Services for Rape Victims: An Application of Multiple Case Study Methodology." *American Journal of Community Psychology* 4, 537-571.

Caraveli, A. 2007. "Building the Future on Member Value: Codevelopment as a Key to Customer Relationships in the 21st Century. *Journal of Association Leadership*.

Carrell, M. R., D. F. Jennings, and C. Heavrin, C. 1997. *Fundamentals of Organizational Behavior*. Upper Saddle River, NJ: Prentice-Hall.

Castelloe, P. 2002. "Participatory Development: Supporting Local Grassroots Efforts." *North Carolina Geographer* 10, 130-135.

CBS News. 2008. "Gap Between Rich and Poor Growing." http://www.cbsnews.com/stories/2008/10/21/business/main4535488.shtml?source=rssat

Ceurstemont, S. 2009. "Revealing the technology of invisibility." Video. *New Scientist*. https://www.Newscientist.com/article/dn16527-video-the-technology-of-invisibility.html

Chan, Z. C. Y., and J. L. C. Ma. 2002. "Anorexic Eating: Two Case Studies in Hong Kong." *The Qualitative Report* 7, no. 4, 24-35.

Chellman, C. C., D. V. Denison, and M. G. Weinstein. 2002. "The Role of Nonprofit Boards in Double Bottom Line Investing." *Journal for Nonprofit Management*, 6, no. 1, 18-30.

Chossudovsky, M. 2008. "Who Are the Architects of Economic Collapse? Will an Obama Administration Reverse the Tide?" *GlobalResearch*. http://www.globalresearch.ca/indexphp?context=vaandaid=10860

Ciuffo, A. 1996. *Characteristics of Successful Entrepreneurs: A Comparison of the Literature with Findings from In-Depth Interviews*. New York: State University of New York, Empire State College.

In *Ethics, the Heart of Leadership*, edited by J. B. Ciulla, 2014. 87-107. Westport, CT: Prager.

Cohen, K. J. and R. M. Cyert. 1965. "Simulation of Organizational Behavior." In *Handbook of Organizations*, edited by J. G. March. Chicago, IL: Rand McNally.

Community-Building in Public Housing: Ties that Bind People and Their Communities. 1997. Washington, DC: The Urban Institute/Aspen Systems Corporation.

Cotton, K. 1994. "Applying Total Quality Management Principles to Secondary Education." http://www.nwrel.org/scpd/ sirs/9/s035.html

Crimm, N. J. 2001. "Private Foundations: Insight for Australia." *Vanderbilt Journal of Transnational Law* 35, 749-799.

Cummings, P. J. 2006. *Beyond Collegiality: Inside the Practice of Systematic Teacher Collaboration in a Public Comprehensive High School.* New York: Columbia University.

Curran, C. J. 2002. "Performance Management: A Help or a Burden to Nonprofits?" *Journal for Nonprofit Management*, 3-19.

Dahl, R. 1999. "Can International Organizations Be Democratic? A Skeptic's View." In *Democracy's Edges*, edited by I. Shapiro and C. Hacker-Cordon, 19-30. Cambridge, UK: Cambridge University Press.

Daniels, S. E. 2006. "Oklahoma School District Goes over the Top." *Quality Progress*, 51-59.

The Deen Show with Eddie, n.d. "Seven Common Questions About Islam." http://www.thedeenshow.com/seven-common-questions-about-islam/

Dees, G. 1998. *The Meaning of Social Entrepreneurship.* Kansas City, MO: Kauffman Center for Entrepreneurial Leadership.

Dennis, R., and B. E. Winston. 2003. "A Factor Analysis of Page and Wong's Servant Leadership Instrument." *Leadership and Organizational Development Journal* 24, no. 8, 455-459.

Deutsch, M. 1985. *Distributive Justice: A Social Psychological Perspective.* New Haven: Yale University Press.

Dobyns, L., and C. Crawford-Mason. 1991. *Quality or Else.* Boston: Houghton Mifflin.

Dunn, M. B. 2006. *Socialization for Innovation: The Role of Developmental Networks.* Boston: Boston College.

Eagly, A, H., M.C. Johannesen-Schmidt, and M. L.Van Eagen. 2003. "Transformal, Transactional and Laissez-Faire Leadership Styles: A Meta-Analysis Comparing Women and Men." *Psychological Bulletin* 129, 567-591.

Emler, N., E. Palmer-Canton, and A. St. James. 1998. "Politics, Moral Reasoning, and the Defining Issues Test: A Reply to Barnett, et al." *British Journal of Social Psychology* 37, 457-476.

Environmental Graffiti. 2008. "Five Deadliest Effects of Global Warming." http://www.environmentalgraffiti.com/sciencetech/5-deadliests-effects-of-global-warming/

Fayol, H. [1919] 1949. *General and Industrial Management.* London: Pitman Publishing.

Fernly-Whittingstall, H. The Observer (Sunday 8, June, 2003). http://www.guardian.co.ub/science/2003/jun/08/gm.food

Fire Department Company Officer, 3rd Ed., (2001. IFSA: Fire Protective Publications Oklahoma.

Fogal, R. E. 2005. "Designing and Managing the Fundraising Program." In *The Jossey-Bass Handbook of Nonprofit Leadership and Management,* 2nd ed., edited by R. D. Herman, 419-435. San Francisco: Jossey Bass.

Follet, M. P. 1949. *Freedom and Co-ordination: Lectures in Business Organizations.* London: Management Publications Trust, Ltd.

Forster, K. 1998. *The Ethics of the Teaching Profession.* Sydney, AU: New South Wales Department of Education and Training.

Fraga, J. 2006. *Affiliation, Empathy and Safety: Perspectives from Students, Teachers, and Principals at Two Small High Schools in New York City.* New York: Columbia University.

Fredriksson, M. 2003. "TQM as a Support for Societal Development." *Total Quality Management* 14, no. 2, 225-233 Freking, K. 2008. "Insurance Gap Leaves Some Elderly to Forgo Medicine: Many in Medicare Stop Treatment When Faced with Paying Full Cost of Prescription." *AP News,* August 21, 2008.

Freed, J. E., M. R. Klugman, and J. D. Fife. 1997. *A Culture for Academic Excellence: Implementing the Quality Principles in Higher Education,* vol. 25. Washington, DC: The George Washington University Graduate School of Education and Human Development.

Freire, P. 1977. *Pedagogy of the Oppressed.* NY: Herder and Herder.

Freire. P. 1985. *The Politics of Education: Culture, Power, and Liberation.* NY: Bergin and Garvey.

Frumkin, M. 2005. *On Being Nonprofit: A Conceptual and Policy Primer.* Cambridge: Harvard University.

Bibliography

Gainer, B., and M. S. Moyer. 2005. "Marketing for Nonprofit Managers." In *The Jossey-Bass Handbook of Nonprofit Leadership and Management*, 2nd ed., edited by R. D. Herman, 277-310. San Francisco: Jossey-Bass.

Gamson, W. A. 1968. *Power and Discontent*. Homewood, IL: Irwin Publications.

Gardner, J. W. 1998. "The American Experiment." *National Civic Review*, 87, no. 3, 193-199.

Garvey, D. G. 2006. *Investigating the Dynamics of Collaboration Experienced by Small, Enterprising Nonprofits*. Storrs: University of Connecticut.

Gazley, B., and J. Brudney. 2007. "The Purpose (and Perils) of Government-Nonprofit Partnership." *Nonprofit and Voluntary Sector Quarterly* 36, no. 3. Los Angeles: Sage Publications.

Giddens, A. 1994. *Beyond Left and Right: The Future of Radical Politics*. Stanford: Stanford University Press.

Gill, H. K. 1999. *The Relationship Between Values and Organizational Commitment: A Multidimensional Perspective*. London: University of Western Ontario.

Gilligan, C. 1982. *In a Different Voice*. Cambridge: Harvard University Press.

Gini, A. 2004. "Moral Leadership and Business Ethics." In *Ethics, The Heart of Leadership,* edited by J. Ciulla, 25-43. Westport, CT: Prager.

Goldberg, J. S., and B. C. Cole. 2002. "Quality Management in Education: Building Excellence and Equity in Student Performance." *Quality Management Journal* 9, no. 4, 3-6

Golden, A. J. March 7, 2000 in a letter to the Honorable Dan Morhaim, Maryland House of Delegates.

Greenleaf Center for Servant Leadership. *Servant Leadership*. www.greenleaf.org/leadership/servant-leadership/what is servant-leadership.html

Guth, W. D., and Ginsberg. 1990. "Corporate Entrepreneurship." *Strategic Management Journal* 11, 11-15.

Habermas, J. 1993. *Moral Consciousness and Communicative Action.* Cambridge, MA: MIT Press.

Haines, G. 1998. *Systems Thinking and Learning.* Amherst, MA: HRD Press.

Haines, G. 2000. *The Systems Thinking Approach to Strategic Planning and Management.* New York: St. Lucie Press.

Hammer, M., and J. Champy. 1993. *Reengineering the Corporation: A Manifesto for Business Revolution.* New York: Harper Business.

Hanieh, A. 2008. "Making the World's Poor Pay: The Economic Crisis and the Global South." https://www.globalresearch.ca/making-the-world-s-poor-pay-the-economic-crisis-and-the-global-south/11100

Hartmann, T. 2004. *Unequal Protection: The Rise of Corporate Dominance and the Theft of Human Rights.* San Francisco, CA: Berrett-Koehler.

Heimbach-Steins, M. 2006. "Education for World Citizens in the Face of Dependency, Insecurity and Loss of Control." *Studies in Christian Ethics* 19, no. 1, 63-80.

Hennigan, P. 2005. *Managing the Introduction of Quality Improvement at Point Park University.* Philadelphia: University of Pennsylvania.

Henderson, A. T., and K. L. Mapp. 2002. *A New Wave of Evidence: The Impact of School, Family, and Community Connections on Student Achievement.* Austin, TX: National Center for Family and Community Connections with Schools, Southwest Educational Laboratory.

Herman, R. D., and R. D. Heimovics. "An Investigation of Leadership Skill Differences in Chief Executives of Nonprofit Organizations." *American Review of Public Administration* 20, 107-124.

History Channel. 2004. "Countdown to Armageddon," December 26, 2004. A and E Television Network.

Holland, T. 2002. "Board Accountability: Lessons from the Field." *Nonprofit Management and Leadership* 12, 409-428.

Hollander, E. P. 2004. "Ethical Challenges in the Leader-Follower Relationship." In *Ethics, the Heart of Leadership,* edited by J. Ciulla, 47-58. Westport, CT: Prager.

Hord, S. M. 1992. *Facilitative Leadership: The Imperative for Change.* Austin, TX: Southwest Educational Development Laboratory.

House, T. J, J. Near, W. Shields, R. Celentano, D. Husband, A. Mercer, and J. Pugh. 1996. *Weather as a Force Multiplier: Owning the Weather in 2025.* http://www.agriculturedefensecoalition.org/sites/default/files/pdfs/5P_1996_U.S._AF2025_v3c15_1_Weather_as_a_Force_Multiplier_Owning_August_1996.pdf

Hradsky, R. D. 2007. *The Conversion of an Upper-Division University to a Four-Year Institution: A Study in Organizational Change.* Philadelphia: University of Pennsylvania.

Hurbert, N. 1987. *Quantum Reality.* New York: Anchor Books.

Hunt, D. V. 1992. *Quality in America: How to Implement a Competitive Quality Program.* Chicago: Irwin Professional Publications.

IRS. 1997. "Publication 557: Tax-exempt Status for Your Organization." Accessed June 2, 2007. http://www.paperglyphs.com/nporegulations/documents/exempt_orgs.html

Irving, J. A. 2005. *Servant Leadership and Effectiveness of Teams.* Virginia Beach, VA: Regent University.

Jeavons, T. H. 2005. "Ethical Nonprofit Management." In *The Jossey-Bass Handbook of Nonprofit Leadership and Management,* 2nd ed., edited by R. D. Herman, 204-230. San Francisco: Jossey-Bass.

Joseph, E. E. 2006. *An Exploration of the Relationship between Servant Leadership Attributes and Leaders' Negotiation Strategy.* Virginia Beach, VA: Regent University.

Joseph, M., and R. Ogletree, R. 1996. "Community Organizing and Comprehensive Community Initiatives." In *Core Issues in Comprehensive Community Building Initiatives,* edited by R. Stone, 3-16. Chicago: Chapin Hall Center for Children.

Katz, J., and J. Mentzos. 1998. *Way to the River Source: A Community's Journey to Supporting Diversity in Schools.* St. Paul, MN: COMPAS, Inc.

Kearney, A. T. 2003. *Waging War on Complexity: How to Master the Matrix Organizational Structure.* San Francisco: CNET Networks, Inc.

Keeley, M. 2004. "The Trouble with Transformational Leadership: Toward a Federalist Ethic for Organizations." *Business Ethics Quarterly* 5, no. 1, 67-96.

Kloos, B., J. McCoy, E. Stewart, E. T. Thomas, A. Wiley, T. L. Good, et al. 1997. "Bridging the Gap: A Community-Based, Open-Systems Approach to School and Neighborhood Consultation." *Journal of Educational and Psychological Consultation* 8, no. 2, 175-196.

Kohlberg, L. 1984. *Essays on Moral Development: The Nature of Validity of Moral Stages, 2*. San Francisco: Harper and Row.

Kotelnikov, V. *Management by Objective*. htt://www.1000ventures.com/ business_guide/mgmt_mbo_html

Kouzes, J. M., and B. Z. Posner. 2003. *Leadership Practices Inventory: Participants' Workbook*. San Francisco: Jossey-Bass Publishers.

Kretzmann, J. P., and J. L. McKnight. 1993. *Building Communities from the Inside Out*. Chicago: Center for Urban Affairs and Policy Research, Northwestern University.

Large, S., A. Macleod, G. Cunningham, and A. Kitson. 2005. *A Multiple-Case Study Evaluation of the RCN Clinical Leadership Programme in England*. London: Royal College of Nursing.

Lee, J. 2001. *Confucian Thought Affecting Leadership and Organizational Culture of Korean Higher Education*. Seoul: Division of Educational Policy Research, Korean Educational Development Institute, Hongik University.

Lewin, K. 1951. *Field Theory in Social Science*. New York: Harper and Row.

Loe, T. W., and W. A. Weeks. 2000. "An Experimental Investigation of Efforts to Improve Sales Students Moral Reasoning." *The Journal of Personal Selling and Sales Management* 20, 243-251.

Lowery, D. 2001. "Implementing Quality Programs in the Nonprofit Sector." *Quality Progress,* 75-80.

Malcolm Baldrige National Quality Award 2000. Gaithersburg, MD: National Institute of Standards and Technology.

Markowitz, L., and K. W. Tice. 2002. "Paradoxes of Professionalization in the Americas." *Gender and Society* 16, no. 6, 941-958.

Maryland Association of Nonprofit Organizations. *1998. Standards for Excellence: An Ethics and Accountability Code for the Nonprofit Sector.* Baltimore: Maryland Association of Nonprofit Organizations.

Maslow, A. H. 1950. *Motivation and Personality.* New York: Harper and Row.

Mattessich, P., and B. Monsey, B. 1997. *Community-Building, What Makes It Work: A Review of Factors Influencing Successful Community-Building.* Saint Paul, MN: Amherst H. Wilder Foundation.

Miller, J. L. 2002. "The Board as Monitor of Organizational Activity: The Applicability of Agency Theory to Nonprofit Boards." *Nonprofit Management and Leadership* 12, 429-450.

Molloy, P., G. Fleming, C. R. Rodriquez, N. Saavedra, B. Tucker, and D. L. Williams. 1995. *Building Home, School, Community Partnerships: The Planning Phase.* Austin, TX: Southwest Educational Development Laboratory.

More, G., and J. A. Whitt. 2000. "Gender and Networks in a Local Voluntary-Sector Elite." *Voluntas* 11, 309-328.

Morely, E., and S. B. Rossman. 1998. *Helping At-Risk Youth.* Washington, DC: The Urban Institute.

Movement Culture. http:/www.wsu.edu:8001/~ a mertu/smc/glossary.html

Moyers, B. 2012. *United States of Alex: Bill Moyers on the secretive corporate-legislative body writing our laws. A special report.* Moyers and Company.

Myers, D. 2001. *BiE . . . Baldrige in Education Initiative: An Innovative Approach for Accelerating School Improvement.* Cincinnati, OH: Hamilton County Educational Service Center.

Naess, A. 1989. *Ecology, Community and Lifestyle: Outline of an Ecosophy,* translated by D. Rothenberg. Cambridge: Cambridge University Press.

National Catholic Register. 2007. *Teacher Abuse Crisis.* http://www.catholic.org/views/views_news.php?id=21030andpid=0

National Community-Building Network. 1998. *An Overview of the National Community- Building Network.* Oakland, CA: National Community-Building Network.

Natural Resources Defense Council. 2016. "Global Warming 101." www.nrdc.org/globalwarming/f101.asp#1

Nunes, T., C. A. Madsen, P. Berus, S. Mlyuer, and A. Nelson. 2002. *Is The Standards of Excellence Making a Difference?* Washington, DC: Aspen Institute.

O'Brien, R. 1998. *An Overview of the Methodological Approach of Action Research.* Toronto: University of Toronto.

Ocshmann, J. L. 2000. *Energy Medicine.* London, UK: Churchill Livingstone.

Oxford Concise Science Dictionary. 1996. s.v. "balance."

Parolini, J. L. 2007. *Investigating the Distinctions between Transformational and Servant leadership.* Virginia Beach, VA: Regent University.

Parsons, T., and R. Bales. 1955. *Family, Socialization and Interaction Process.* Glencoe, IL: The Free Press.

Patel, R. 2002. "The Profits of Famine: Southern Africa's Long Decade of Hunger." http://www.thirdworldtraveler.com/Africa/Profits_Famine.html

Patton, M. Q. 1981. *Practical Evaluation.* Beverly Hills, CA: Sage Publications.

Patton, M. Q. 1990. *Qualitative Evaluation and Research.* Newbury Park, CA: Sage Publications.

Patton, M. Q. 1997. *Utilization-Focused Evaluation: The New Century Text,* 3rd ed. Thousand Oaks, CA: Sage Publications.

Pellow, J. P. 2006. *The Impact of Leadership on Institutional Culture and Mission: A Case Study of St. John's University, 1989-2005.* Philadelphia: University of Pennsylvania.

Perkins, J. 2007. *The Secret History of the American Empire.* New York: Penguin.

Perkins, M. D. 2007. *The Dynamics of Leadership and Change at Three Small Colleges.* Philadelphia: University of Pennsylvania.

Peters, B. G. 1998. "With a Little Help from Our Friends: Public-Private Partnerships as Institutions and Instruments." In *Partnerships in Urban Governance*, edited by J. Pierre, 11-33. New York: St. Martin's Press.

Peters, F. E. 1990. *Judaism, Christianity and Islam: The Classical Texts and Their Interpretations, vol. I: The World and the Law and the People of God*. Princeton, NJ: Princeton University Press.

Pinchot, G. 1985. *Intrapreneuring: Why You Don't Have to Leave the Corporation to Become an Entrepreneur*. New York: Harper and Row.

Pollak, T. 2007. *The Nonprofit Sector in Brief: Facts and Figures from the Nonprofit Almanac*. Washington, DC: Urban Institute.

Posner, P. L. (2002. "Accountability Challenges of Third Sector Government." In *The Tools of Government*, edited by L. M. Salamon, 523-551. New York: Oxford University Press.

Prichavudhi, A. 2003. *School Leaders Perspectives on Effective Change in a Thai Catholic School through Systems Thinking: A Case Study*. Philadelphia: University of Pennsylvania.

Quinn, R., and J. Rohrbaugh. 1983. "A Spatial Model of Effectiveness Criteria: Towards A Competing Values Approach to Organizational Analysis." *Management Science* 29, 363-377.

Reader's Digest Great Encyclopedic Dictionary. 1973. s.v. "evolution."

Reid, E. J., editor. 1998. *Nonprofit and Government: Collaboration and Conflict*. Washington, DC: The Urban Institute.

Reid, E. J. 2000. *Understanding the Word Advocacy: Context and Use*. Washington, DC: The Urban Institute.

Rest, J. R., and D. Narvaez. 1998. *DIT-2: The Defining Issues Test*. Minneapolis: University of Minnesota Center for Research in Ethical Development.

Roberts, J. 2007. "Is Russia Preparing for World War III? Secrets of Survival." http://www.secrets of survival.com/survival/is _russia _preparing _for_war.html

Robinson, C. C. 2004. *Women in High School Principalships: A Comparison of Four Case Studies from a Virginia Public School District from 1970-2000*. Falls Church: Virginia Polytechnic Institute and State University.

Roderiquez, S. A. 2007. *Outrageous Leadership: Three Exemplary Principals and the Climate They Create*. Philadelphia: University of Pennsylvania.

Rosenblum, N. 1998. *Membership and Morals: The Personal Uses of Pluralism in America*. Princeton, NJ: Princeton University.

Russell, R. F. 2000. *Exploring the Values and Attributes of Servant Leaders*. Virginia Beach, VA: Regent University.

Salamon, L. M. 2002. "The New Governance and the Tools of Public Action: An Introduction." In *The Tools of Government*, edited by L. M. Salamon, 1-47. New York: Oxford University Press.

Salem, D., P. Foster-Fishman, and J. Goodkind. 1999. *The Adoption of Innovation in Not-For-Profit Advocacy Organizations*. Washington, DC: Aspen Institute.

Schein, E. H. 2004. *Organizational Culture and Leadership*, 3d ed. San Francisco: Jossey-Bass.

Schneider, B. 1987. "The People Make the Place." *Personnel Psychology* 40, 437-453.

Schneider, S. K., and G. B. Northcraft. 1999. "Three Social Dilemmas of Workforce Diversity in Organizations: A Social Identity Perspective." *Human Relations* 52, 1445-1467.

Schwartz, S. H. 1996. "Value Priorities and Behavior: Applying a Theory of Integrated Values Systems." In *The Ontario Symposium* 8, edited by C. Seligman and J. M. Olsen, 1-24.

Schwartz, S. H., and W. Bilsky. 1987. "Toward a Universal Psychological Structure of Human Values." *Journal of Personality and Social Psychology* 53, no. 3, 550-562.

Sciaraffa, M. 2004. *Profiles of Early Childhood Education Administrators: Looking for Patterns of Leadership*. Baton Rouge: Louisiana State University.

Scope, P. S. 2006. *Relationship between Leadership Styles of Middle School Principals and School Culture*. West Lafayette, IN: Purdue University.

Senge, P. M. 1994. *The Fifth Discipline: The Art and Practice of The Learning Organization*. New York: Currency Doubleday.

Sevastopulo, D. 2005. "U.S. Nuclear Weapons Parts Missing, Pentagon Says." *Financial Times* http://www.ft.com/ems/s/0/04dfa24c-3dbg-11dd-bbb5-0000779fd2ac.html?nclick_check=l

Sgro, A. H. 2006. *The Perception of Parents of the Appropriate Degree of Parent Involvement in an Independent Boarding School: A Matter of Trust*. Philadelphia: Pennsylvania University.

Shirk, A. O. 2006. *Co-Activity as Leading and Learning: Emergence of Leadership from Presence to Interrelationship*. NY: Columbia University.

Slavinsky, R. A. 2006. *Cognitive Moral Development of Connecticut Public School Principals as Measured by Rest's Defining Issues Test*. Storrs: University of Connecticut.

Smith, A. [1776] 2003. *The Wealth of Nations*. New York: Bantam Books.

Solomon, R. C. 2004. "Ethical Leadership, Emotions, and Trust: Beyond 'Charisma'." In *Ethics the Heart of Leadership*, 2nd ed., edited by J. B. Ciulla, 83-102. Westbury, CT: Quorum Books

Srivastva, A. "In Search of Noble Organizing: A Study in Social Entrepreneurship." PhD dissertation, Case Western Reserve University, 2004. https://etd.ohiolink.edu/pg_10?0::NO:10:P10_ACCESSION_NUM:case1081265383

Stake, R. E. 1995. *The Art of Case Study Research*. Thousand Oaks, CA: Sage Publications.

Stevens, S. K. 2003. *In Their Own Words: The Entrepreneurial Behavior of Nonprofit Founders*. Cincinnati, OH: The Graduate School of the Union Institute and University.

Stone, M. M., and F. Ostrower. 2007. "Acting in The Public Interest? Another Look at Research on Nonprofit Governance." *Nonprofit Voluntary Sector Quarterly* 36, no. 3, 416-438.

Su, C. 2005. *Streetwise for Book Smarts: Culture, Community Organizing, and Education Reform in the Bronx*. Boston: Massachusetts Institute of Technology.

Sylvia, R. D., and K. M. Sylvia. 2004. *Program Planning and Evaluation for the Public Manager*. Long Grove, IL: Waveland Press.

Taylor, A. T. 2006. *Questioning Participation: Critical Policy Scholarship and Education Reform in Tanzania*. NY: Columbia University.

Tellis, W. 1997. "Introduction to Case Study." *The Qualitative Report* 3, no. 2.

Tischler, L. 2005. "God and Mammon at Harvard." *Fast Company Magazine*, 47-54.

Tishler, C. 2001. "Enterprising Nonprofits: A Toolkit for Social Entrepreneurs - Why Running a Nonprofit is the Hardest Job in Business." http://hbswk.hbs.edu/archive/2265.html

Tobias, L. L. 1990. "Selecting for Excellence: How to Hire the Best." *Nonprofits World* 8, no. 2, 23-25.

U.S. Charter Schools. http://www.uscharterschools.org/pub/uscs_docs/0/index.

Van Engen, M. L., R. van der Leeden, and T. M. Willemsen. 2001. "Gender, Context and Leadership Styles: A Field Study." *Journal of Occupational Organizational Psychology* 74, 581-598.

Van Maanen, J., and T. Barley. 1985. "Cultural Organizations: Fragments of a Theory." In *Organizational Culture*, edited by P. J. Frost, L. F. Moore, M. R. Louis, C.C. Lundberg, and J. Martin, 31-54. Beverly Hills, CA: Sage Publishing.

VanSandt, C.V. 2001. *An Examination of the Relationship between Ethical Work Climate and Moral Awareness*. Blacksburg: Virginia Polytechnic Institute and State University.

Victor, B., and J. B. Cullen. 1988. "The Organizational Bases of Ethical Work Climates." *Administrative Science Quarterly* 33, 101-125.

Vogelsang, J. D. 1998. "Values-Based Organizational Development." *Journal for Nonprofit Management* 2, no. 1, 12-17.

Vogelsang, J. D. 2002. "We Are on Our Way: A Continuous Change Approach to Organizational Development." *Journal for Nonprofit Management* 6, no. 1, 35-47.

Vogt, W. P., 1993. *Dictionary of Statistics and Methodology: A Nontechnical Guide for the Social Sciences*. Thousand Oaks, CA: Sage Publications.

Wagner, C. 2005. "Leadership for an Improved School Culture: How to Assess and Improve the Culture of Your School." *Kentucky School Leader,* 1-3.

Walton, J. 2002. *The Characteristics of the Organization Culture of Six Effective Substance Abuse Programs: An Exploratory Study.* Santa Barbara, CA: Fielding Graduate Institute.

Warwick, M. 2000. *The Five Strategies of Fundraising Success: A Mission-Based Guide to Achieving Your Goals.* San Francisco: Jossey-Bass Publishers.

Weathers, J. M. 2006. *A Multilevel Organizational Analysis of the Effects of School Policies and Leadership on Teacher Community in Urban Elementary Schools.* Philadelphia: University of Pennsylvania.

Webber, J. B. 2003. *How Can Action Research Help a Nonprofit Develop and Position Itself to Become More Valuable and Relevant.* Santa Barbara, CA: Fielding Graduate Institute.

Weber, J. 1995. "Influences upon Organizational Ethical Subclimates: A Multi-Departmental Analysis of a Single Firm." *Organizational Science 6,* 503-523.

Weber, M. [1905] 1958. *The Protestant Ethic and the Spirit of Capitalism,* translated by T. Parsons. New York: Scribner's Sons.

Weber, M. 1954. *Max Weber on Law, Economy and Society.* Cambridge, MA: Harvard University Press.

Weber, M. 1968. *Economy and Society.* New York: Bedminster Press.

Wehlage, G., R. Rutter, and C. Stone. 1986. *Wisconsin Youth Survey.* Madison, WI: National Center on Effective Secondary Schools.

Weiss, W. et al. 2005. "Problematic Police Performance and Personality Assessment Inventory." *Journal of Police and Criminal Psychology.*

Wheelen, T. L., and S. D. Hunger. 2002. *Strategic Management and Business Policy.* Upper Saddle River, NJ: Prentice Hall.

Wies, J. R. 2006. *The Changing Relationships of Women Helping Women: Patterns and Trends in Domestic Violence Advocacy.* Lexington: University of Kentucky.

Willett, W. N. 2006. *The Cultural Impact of the Frontieri Myth and the Protestant Ethic on Principal Leadership and Their Influence on Teacher Commitment.* Storrs: University of Connecticut.

Xu, Q. 2007. "Community Participation in China: Identifying Mobilization Factors." *Nonprofit Voluntary Sector Quarterly* 36, no. 4, 622-642.

Yin, R. 1994. *Case Study Research: Design and Methods*, 2nd ed.. Beverly Hills, CA: Sage Publishing.

Young, D. R. 1986. "Entrepreneurship and the Behavior of Nonprofit Organizations: Elements of a Theory." In *The Economics of Nonprofit Institutions: Studies in Structure and Policy,* edited by S. Rose-Ackerman. New York: Oxford University Press.

Zucker, D. M. 2001. "Using Case Study Methodology in Nursing Research." *The Qualitative Report* 6, no. 2, 32-41.

CPSIA information can be obtained
at www.ICGtesting.com
Printed in the USA
FSHW021445230320
68385FS